FATTY LIVER DIET COOKBOOK

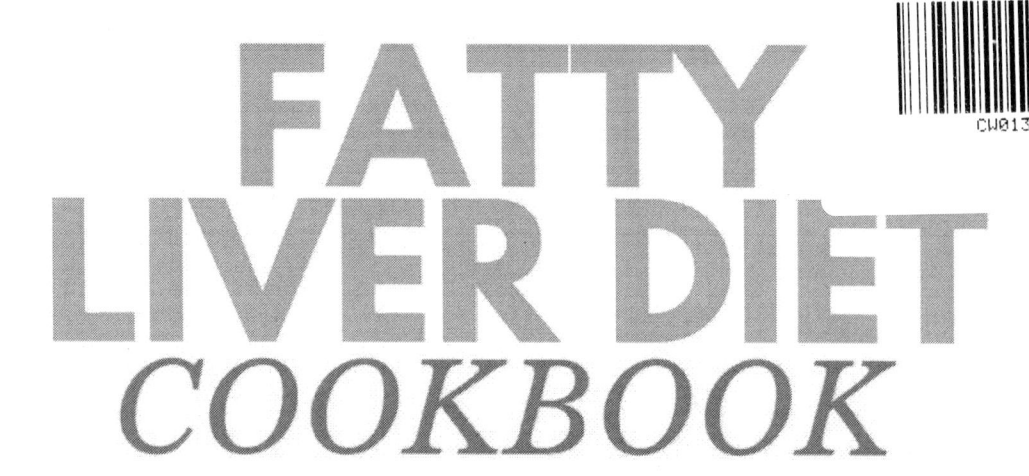

Give Your Liver a Push in the Right Direction by Making the Switch to Healthy, Delicious Recipes and a Liver-Friendly Diet

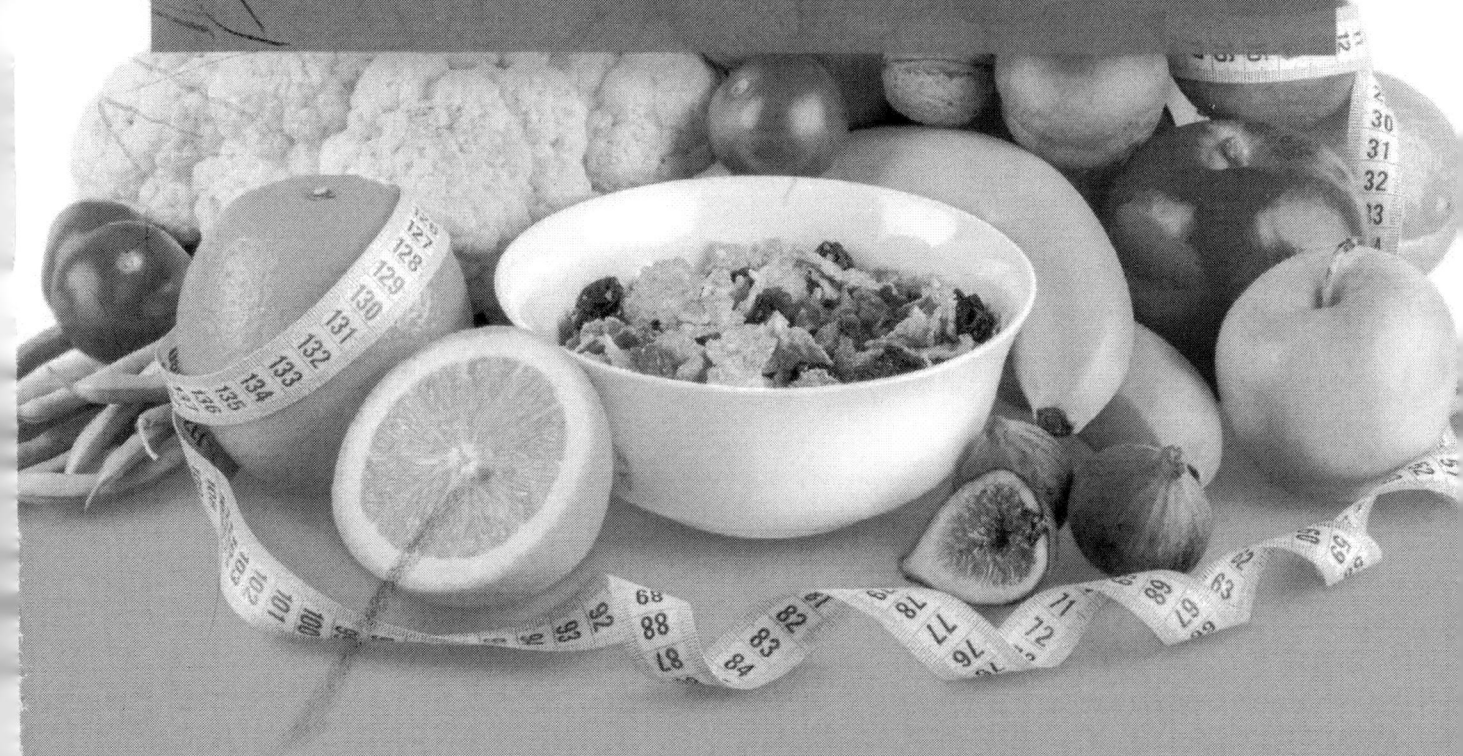

© **Copyright 2022 - All rights reserved.**

The content contained within this book may not be reproduced, duplicated or transmitted without direct written permission from the author or the publisher.

Under no circumstances will any blame or legal responsibility be held against the publisher, or author, for any damages, reparation, or monetary loss due to the information contained within this book, either directly or indirectly.

Legal Notice:

This book is copyright protected. It is only for personal use. You cannot amend, distribute, sell, use, quote or paraphrase any part, or the content within this book, without the consent of the author or publisher.

Disclaimer Notice:

Please note the information contained within this document is for educational and entertainment purposes only. All effort has been executed to present accurate, up to date, reliable, complete information. No warranties of any kind are declared or implied. Readers acknowledge that the author is not engaged in the rendering of legal, financial, medical or professional advice. The content within this book has been derived from various sources. Please consult a licensed professional before attempting any techniques outlined in this book.

By reading this document, the reader agrees that under no circumstances is the author responsible for any losses, direct or indirect, that are incurred as a result of the use of the information contained within this document, including, but not limited to, errors, omissions, or inaccuracies.

Table of Contents

Introduction 2
Chapter 1 About the Liver, Functions, etc. 4
   Functions of the Liver 4
   Fatty Liver Diseases 5
Chapter 2 Guidelines for a Forever Healthy Liver 9
   Foods to Eat and Avoid 11
   Health Benefits of Various Foods 12
Chapter 3: Breakfast 15
   Cherry Berry Bulgur Bowl 16
   Baked Curried Apple Oatmeal Cups 16
   Healthy Millet Porridge 17
   Peanut Butter and Cacao Breakfast Quinoa ... 17
   Egg and Veggie Muffins 18
   Breakfast Tacos 18
   Vegetable Omelet 19
   Buckwheat and Grapefruit Porridge 19
   Raspberry Pudding 20
   Pineapple, Macha & Beet Chia Pudding 20
   Tapioca Pudding 21
   Banana Pancakes 21
   Nectarine Pancakes 22
   Pancakes 22
   Peach Muffins 23
   Blueberry Muffins 23
   Avocado Spread 24
   Deviled eggs 24
   Spicy Cucumbers 25
   Herbed Spinach Frittata 25
   Pumpkin Flax Granola 26
   Broiled Parmesan Avocado 26
   Mexican Scrambled Eggs in Tortilla 27
   Raspberry Overnight Porridge 27
   Turkey and Spinach Scramble on Melba Toast 28
   Mexican Style Burritos 28
   Quinoa Bowls With Avocado and Egg 29
Chapter 4: Vegetarian Mains 30
   Tofu Rice 31
   Green Buddha Bowl 31
   Tofu Spinach Sauté 32
   Roasted Green Beans and Mushrooms 32
   Vegetable and Egg Casserole 33
   Zucchini Boat 33
   Zucchini Cups 34
   Easy Asparagus Quiche 34
   Balsamic Mushroom and Asparagus 35
   Crunchy Quinoa Meal 35
   Pasta With Indian Lentils 36
   Cranberry and Roasted Squash Delight 36
   Mozzarella Pasta Mix 37
   Citrus Quinoa & Chickpea Salad 37
   Rosemary Roasted New Potatoes 38
   Couscous and Toasted Almonds 38
   Chickpeas and Beets Mix 39
   Air Fryer Stuffed Peppers 39
   Avocado Boat with Salsa 40
   Low-Carb Berry Salad With Citrus Dressing .. 40
   Spaghetti Squash 41
   Zucchini and Tomatoes 41
   Vegan Meatballs 42
   Spinach Alfredo Soup 42
   Air Fryer Spaghetti Squash 43
   Asparagus With Garlic 43
   Zucchini Lasagna 44
   Mexican Cauliflower Rice 44

Quick Collard Greens 45

Chapter 5: Grains, Beans, and Legumes 46

Black Eyed Peas Stew 47
Chickpea Alfredo Sauce 47
Chickpea Eggplant Salad 48
Extraordinary Green Hummus 48
Bell Peppers 'N Tomato-Chickpea Rice 49
Spaghetti in Lemon Avocado White Sauce 49
Kidney Beans and Beet Salad 50
Kidney Beans and Parsley-lemon Salad 50
Italian White Bean Soup 51
Sicilian-Style Zoodle Spaghetti 51
Tasty Lime Cilantro Cauliflower Rice 52
Fennel Wild Rice Risotto 52
Wild Rice Prawn Salad 53
White Bean Soup 53
Black Bean Hummus 54
Brussels Sprouts 'N White Bean Medley 54
Chicken and White Beans 55
Cilantro-Dijon Vinaigrette on Kidney Beans Salad 55
Chickpea Salad Moroccan Style 56
White Bean Smoothie to Burn Fats 56

Chapter 6: Beef, Pork, and Lamb 57

Hot Pork Meatballs 59
Tasty Lamb Ribs 59
Beef Spread 60
Pork Chops and Relish 60
Lamb and Tomato Sauce 61
Lemony Lamb and Potatoes 61
Cumin Lamb Mix 62
Pork and Figs Mix 62
Greek Style Lamb Chops 63
Pork and Peas 63
Pork and Sage Couscous 64
Pork Fajitas 64
Apple Spice Pork Chops 65

Beef Burritos 65

Chapter 7: Poultry 66

Oven Roasted Garlic Chicken Thigh 67
Grilled Harissa Chicken 67
Italian Chicken Meatballs 68
Classic Chicken Cooking With Tomatoes & Tapenade 68
Grilled Grapes & Chicken Chunks 69
Turkish Turkey Mini Meatloaves 69
Lemon Caper Chicken 70
Herb Roasted Chicken 70
Grilled Chicken Breasts 71
Turkey Meatballs 71
Chicken Marsala 72
Lean and Green Chicken Pesto Pasta 72
Chicken Stuffed Peppers 73
Turkey Fritters and Sauce 73
Herbed Chicken Stew 74
Grilled Chicken 74
Turkey With Leeks and Radishes 75
Turkey and Cranberry Sauce 75
Coconut Chicken 76
Ginger Chicken Drumsticks 76
Pomegranate Chicken 77
Lemon Chicken Mix 77
Cardamom Chicken and Apricot Sauce 78
Chicken and Spinach Cakes 78
Chicken and Parsley Sauce 79
Chicken Marsala -day10: italian white bean soup 79
Curry Chicken, Artichokes, and Olives 80
Vegetable Ribbon Noodles with Chicken Breast Fillet 80
Zucchini and Mozzarella Casserole 81
Herby Chicken Meatloaf 81

Chapter 8: Fish and Seafood 82

Tilapia with Avocado & Red Onion 83

Herbed Roasted Cod................................. 83	Detox-Liver Arugula and Broccoli Soup........102
Smoked Salmon and Watercress Salad............ 84	Unique Lentil With Kale Soup 103
Salmon and Corn Salad 84	Pasta Veggies Minestrone Soup 103
Feta and Pesto Wrap 85	Zucchini Noodles Soup 104
Salmon Bowls... 85	Chicken Oatmeal Soup...................................104
Salmon with Vegetables 86	Celery Cream Soup 105
Salmon Burgers 86	Mint Quinoa 105
Black Cod 87	Pear Red Pepper Soup 106
Miso-Glazed Salmon.................................. 87	Low Heat Chicken Provençal 106
Niçoise Salad 88	Danny's Tortellini Soup 107
Baked Fish With Feta and Tomato 88	Wellness Parsnip Soup 107
Salmon Panatela 89	Feel Good Chicken Soup................................108
Shrimp Fried "Rice" 89	Pork Soup..108
Barbecued Spiced Tuna With Avocado-Mango Salsa... 90	Curry Soup..109
Salmon Foil-Pack 90	Yellow Onion Soup..109
Yummy Cedar Planked Salmon 91	Garlic Soup..110
Quick Delicious Maple Salmon 91	**Chapter 10: Salads 111**
Pan Seared Salmon 92	Cauliflower Salad 112
Lemon Rosemary Salmon 92	Avocado Tomato Salad 112
Crispy Fish 93	Crispy Fennel Salad 113
Tuna Noodle Casserole 93	Arugula and Sweet Potato Salad 113
Seared Scallops 94	Provencal Summer Salad 113
Salmon Pasta 94	Bean and Toasted Pita Salad...........................114
Crusty Pesto Salmon.................................. 95	Beans and Spinach Mediterranean Salad.......114
Sesame Tuna Steak.................................... 95	Spring Greens Salad 115
Foil Packet Lobster Tail 96	Tuna Salad...115
Chapter 9: Soups and Stews 97	Fish Salad 115
Grilled Tomatoes Soup 98	Salmon Salad...116
Lean Mean Soup 98	Arugula Salad with Shallot.............................116
Crockpot Lentil Soup................................. 99	Roasted Bell Pepper Salad with Anchovy Dressing..116
Turmeric Chicken Soup 99	Roasted Vegetable Salad................................117
Healthy Silky Tortilla Soup 100	Spanish Tomato Salad 117
Healthy Carrot Ginger Soup........................... 100	Grilled Salmon Summer Salad 117
Chicken Tortilla Avocado Soup 101	Garden Salad With Oranges and Olives 118
Spicy Chicken and Kale 101	Salmon & Arugula Salad 118
Halibut Tomato Soup 102	Farro Salad 119

Carrot Salad 119
Beets Steamed Edamame Salad 119
Avocado Cilantro Chunky Salsa 120
Toasted Mango Pepitas Kale Salad 120
Chickpeas and Parsley Pumpkin Salad 121
Springtime Chicken Berries Salad.................. 121
Toaster Almond Spiralized Beet Salad 122
Eggplant Garlic Salad with Tomatoes 122

Chapter 11: Desserts 123
Honey-Cinnamon Grilled Plums................... 124
Lemon Ricotta Peaches................................... 124
Rhubarb Compote... 124
Grilled Pineapple Strips.................................. 125
Nutmeg Lemon Pudding................................ 125
Fruit Medley.. 126
Lemon and Semolina Cookies........................ 126
Semolina Cake 127
Banana Kale Smoothie.................................... 127
Lime Grapes and Apples 128
Apple Crisp 128
Strawberry and Avocado Medley................... 129
Watermelon Ice Cream 129
Raspberry Walnut Sorbet 130

Chapter 12: Juice and Smoothie (Specific for Liver Health).. 131
Breakfast Smoothie 132
Clean Liver Green Juice.................................. 132
Green Tea Purifying Smoothie....................... 132
Blue Breeze Shake... 133
Fats Burning & Water Based Smoothies........ 133
Smoothie with Ginger and Cucumber 134
Oatmeal Blast with Fruit 134
White Bean Smoothie to Burn Fats 134
Meal Replacement Smoothie with Banana ... 135
Coconut Cherry Smoothie 135
Grapes and Peach Smoothie 135
Twin Berry Smoothie...................................... 136

Light Fiber Smoothie 136
Peach and Kiwi Smoothie 136
Cashew Boost Smoothie 137
Heavy Metal Cleansing Smoothie..................137
Power Detox Smoothie....................................138
Detox Action Super Green Smoothie.............138
Kale Batch Detox Smoothie 139
Smoothie with A Spirit 139
Alkaline Green Bliss Smoothie.......................140
Smooth Root Green Cleansing Smoothie......140
Glory Smoothie 141
Strawberry Nutty Smoothie...........................141
Tropical Green Tea 141
Old Spice Ginger Tea......................................142
Healthy Vacation Peach Drink.......................142

Chapter 13: 28-Day Meal Plan to Detox the Liver 143

Measurement Conversion Chart............... 146
Volume Equivalents (Liquid) 146
Volume Equivalents (Dry)..............................146
Oven Temperatures 147
Weight Equivalents 148

Conclusion... 149

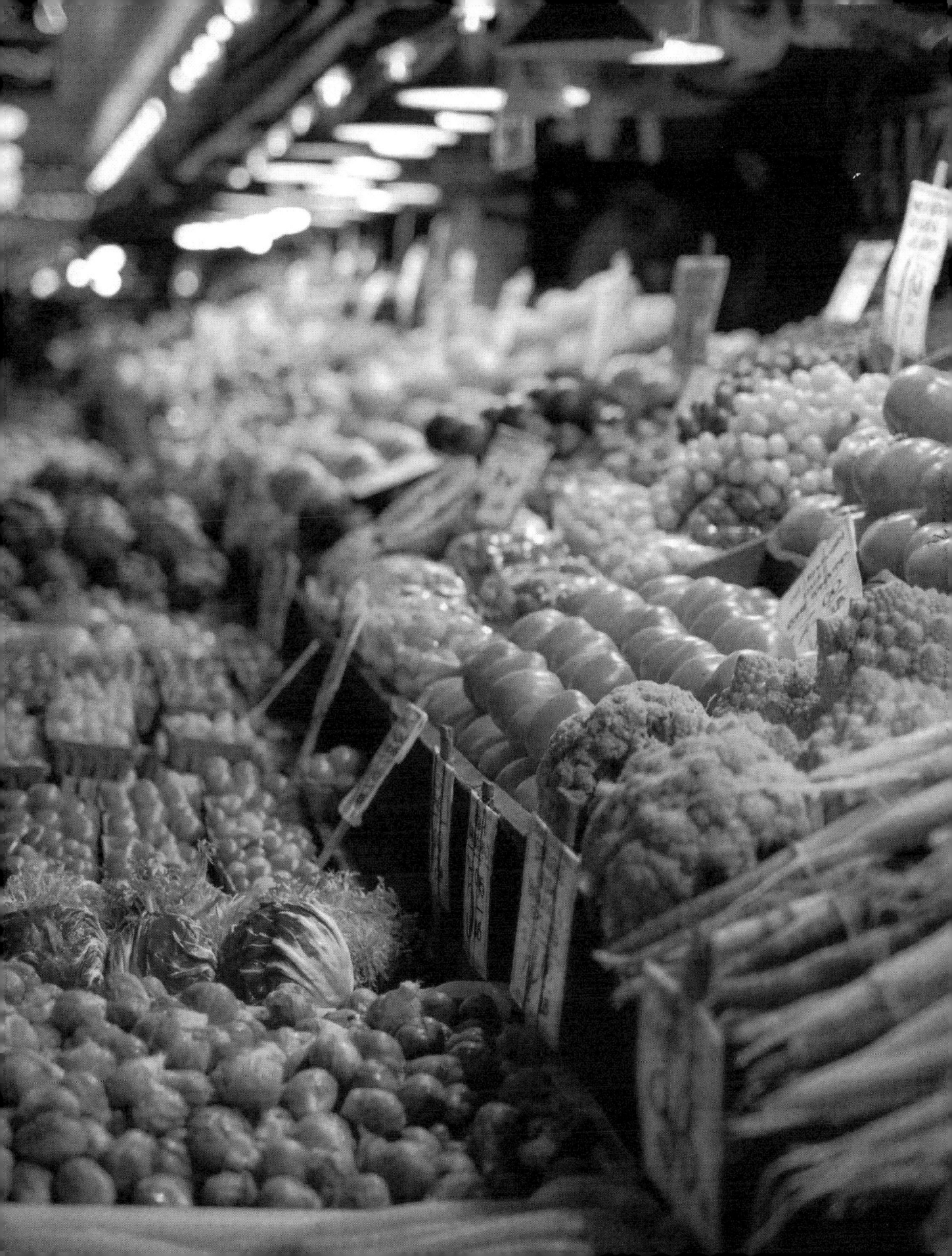

Introduction

You're probably reading this book because you or a loved one has been diagnosed with fatty liver or steatosis. As physicians, we want you to know you're in good company. Fatty liver is a health problem that's increasing in frequency, partially due to lifestyle choices and a rise in the number of obese people. About a third of the population has fatty liver disease. Surprised?

Fatty liver is more common than another common liver problem you hear more about, viral hepatitis. This disease hasn't gotten the attention it deserves and that's unfortunate since it can negatively impact your health.

Many people have the condition but are not necessarily aware of it until they start suffering from symptoms and are formally diagnosed with liver damage. People can live with a fatty liver without knowing it for a long time, but at some point, they may experience an inflamed liver. Approximately 20 to 25% of individuals with NASH will progress to cirrhosis, a serious health problem where the liver becomes scarred and loses the ability to function normally.

By managing your food consumption, you can, in turn, manage the effects of a fatty liver. This will improve your lifestyle, one in which symptoms have a less direct impact on your life, and any pain can become more manageable. With this diet cookbook, you can start losing weight correctly and gain nutritional value from food which will make it easier to monitor your cholesterol and will hopefully inspire you to be more active. The reality is: How we choose to feed our bodies can impact us suddenly or much later in our life.

By choosing to invest in this diet cookbook, you will expand your knowledge regarding what foods to consume that have the best nutritional value and learn how they will impact your life, helping you make better meal choices.

If you have recently been diagnosed with fatty liver disease, you might now be faced with many questions, and you may be looking back thinking, "I should have made smarter choices with what I was consuming…" You can make the necessary changes today to improve your life quality.

Enjoying meals that are prepared to assist you with maintaining and managing your symptoms and consuming food high in nutritional benefits that can optimize liver functions will result in allowing you to enjoy a healthier lifestyle to the fullest. Medicate yourself with food! Prioritizing your health has never been easier than in this diet cookbook. If you are ready, join us in living a healthier life.

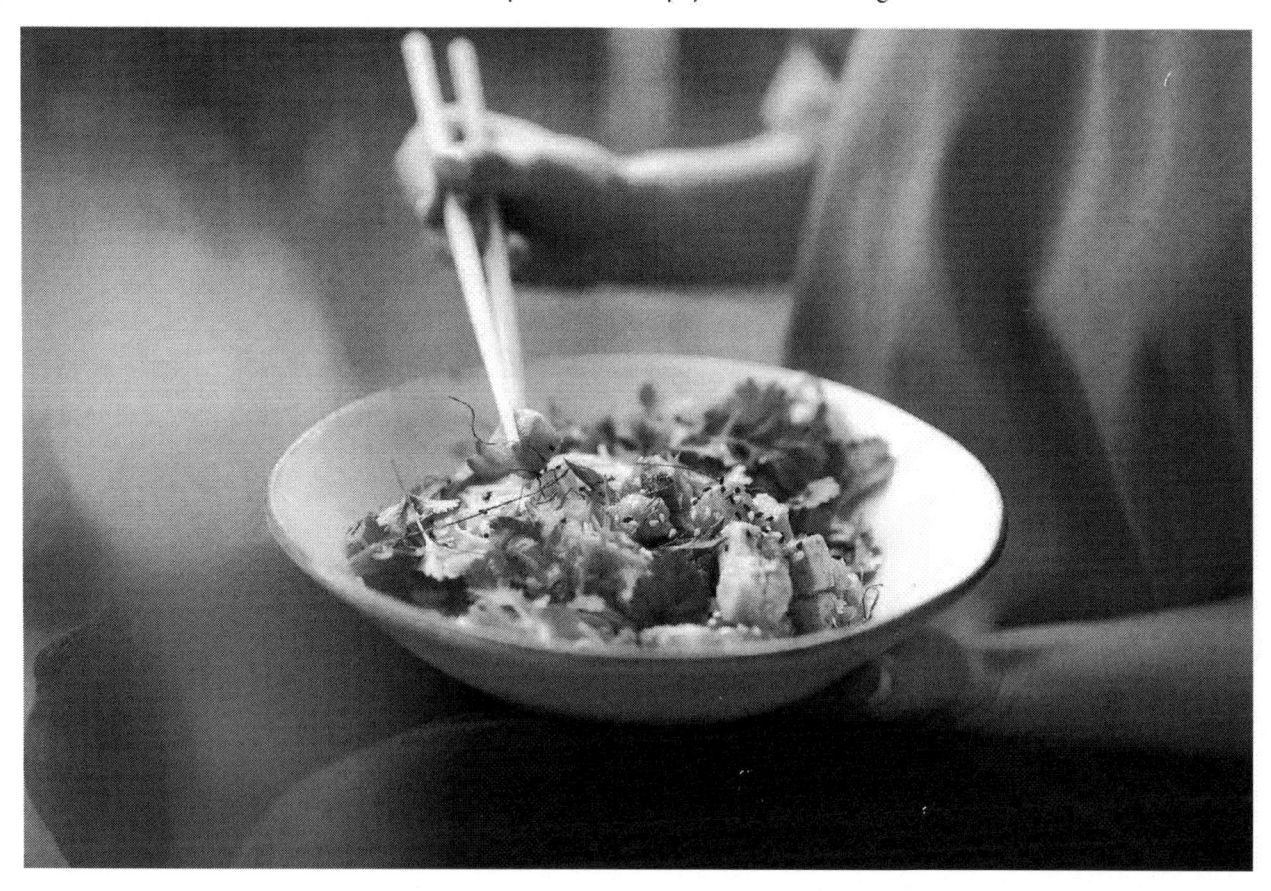

Chapter 1

About the Liver, Functions, etc.

Functions of the Liver

In general, the liver has approximately 500 different functions. Some of its important functions are listed below:

- Processing the food once it has been digested.
- Cleaning and filtering the blood.
- Producing bile that aids the digestion of lipids in the small intestine.
- Maintaining and producing hormone balance in our body.
- Producing proteins and enzymes that aid in chemical reactions in the body, for example, blood clotting and repairing tissue.
- Safeguarding us by fighting infections and diseases.
- Destroying and dealing with harmful chemicals such as drugs or poisons.
- Helping in controlling cholesterol.
- Storing and releasing a tremendous amount of energy that can be used rapidly when the body needs it most.
- Storing minerals, vitamins, sugars, and iron.
- The greatest of all is that our liver repairs its damage and renews itself.

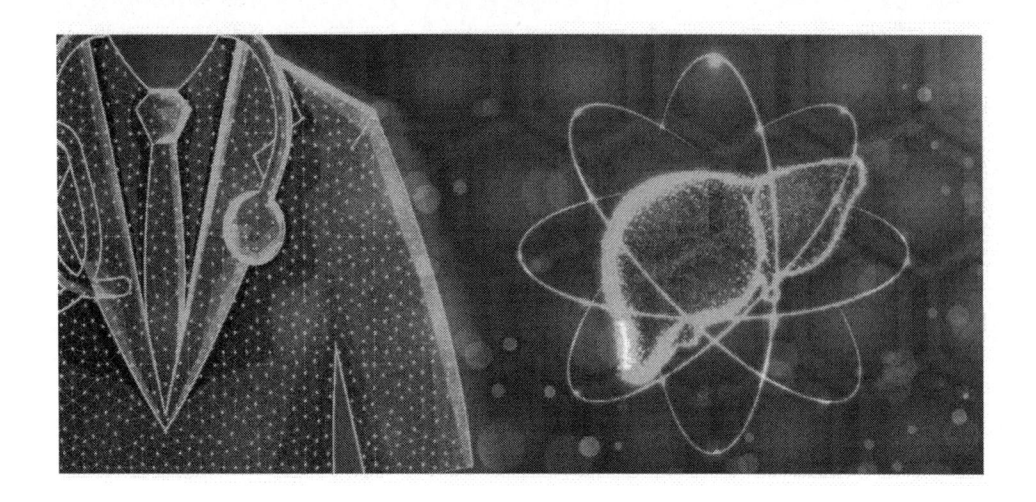

Fatty Liver Diseases

Various illnesses can affect the liver, including, but not limited to:

Liver Failure

When you have liver failure, it means that your liver has lost most, if not all, of its liver function, a serious condition that requires emergency medical attention. The first symptoms you will notice are diarrhea, extreme nausea, fatigue, and a loss of appetite. Because these symptoms are common to many other ailments your body could be suffering from, it can be difficult to know that your liver is failing.

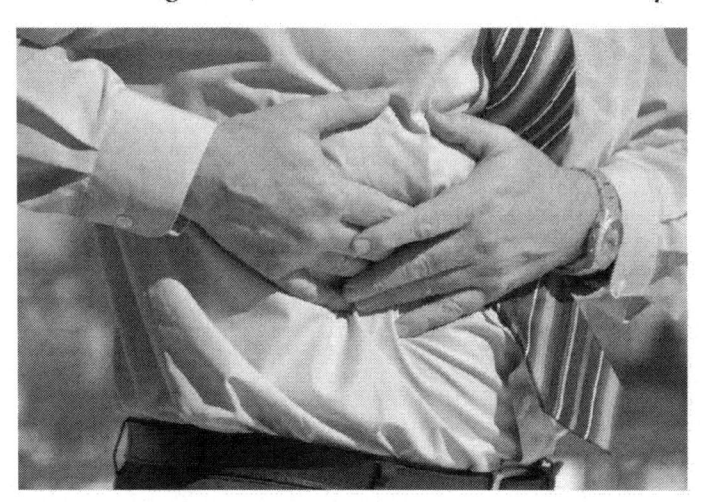

However, as liver failure becomes more and more advanced, the symptoms continue advancing too, and the patient may start getting disoriented, confused, and unusually sleepy. If unattended to, there is a very high risk of coma or death in the worst-case scenario. Doctors will try to save any part of the liver that is still working; if this is impossible, the other option will be a transplant.

In an event of liver failure due to cirrhosis, it means that the patient's liver has been gradually getting sicker and failing over time, possibly for several years, and is referred to as chronic liver failure or End

Stage Liver Disease. Although very rare, liver failure could also be caused by malnutrition. Acute liver failure is when liver failure is very sudden, occurs in as little as two days, and is usually caused by a medication overdose or a severe case of poisoning.

Liver Cancer

It is important to note that cancer in the liver can progress at any stage of liver disease, and that's why routine checkups are very important as they make it possible to catch cancer, if any, at a very early stage that's removable before it progresses to the entire liver.

Alcoholic Liver Disease (ALD)

If you are a heavy drinker or have been drinking alcohol excessively, this is the first stage of injury to your liver due to the buildup of fatty deposits. If proper care is taken and you stay away from alcohol, this can be completely reversed. As per the studies, only 20% of people with alcohol-related fatty liver go on to develop inflammation (alcoholic hepatitis) and eventually cirrhosis.

People who have been drinking alcohol excessively and have alcoholic liver damage have been found mostly malnourished, which means their body lacks the nutrients that it requires to function properly. This lack of nourishment could be due to several factors; some common ones are:

- If you are not eating well and just drinking, you are asking your body to work hard to process alcohol. Alcohol has no nutritional value but requires a lot of energy for the body to process.
- Poor or un-balanced diet.
- Loss of appetite due to heavy drinking. If you are drinking and smoking, the condition will worsen. Smoking is known for suppressing hunger.
- Poor absorption of food nutrients as the liver is less able to produce bile to aid digestion.

You could be undernourished even if you are overweight. It all depends on what and how you eat. If you eat well and still becoming overweight, get yourself checked, if not already. This condition could be due to fluid retention.

You should be prescribed Vitamin B if you have been drinking excessively or at harmful levels. People with alcoholic liver disease generally lack the vitamin called thiamin, a vitamin B that helps the body convert carbohydrates into energy. Consult your doctor or dietitian if this has not been prescribed.

N.A.F.L.D - Non-Alcoholic Fatty Liver Disease

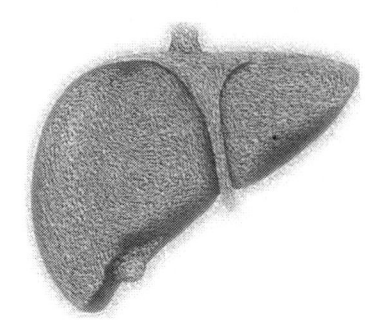

As the name suggests, non-alcoholic fatty liver disease is a condition when there is a fat buildup in the liver cells even if the patient does not drink alcohol excessively. At the initial stages, the fat deposits may not trigger any symptoms, but it has been found that in some cases, this may progress to inflammation called Nonalcoholic Steatohepatitis (NASH), which can further lead to scarring of the tissues in the liver and even cirrhosis.

People may still develop a fatty liver without excessive consumption of alcohol. There could be several factors for developing a fatty liver. Your likelihood of developing fatty liver conditions is higher if you:

- Have diabetes.
- Are obese or overweight.
- Have an insulin-resistance body; your body does not respond to insulin as it should.
- Have high levels of cholesterol.

You may be advised to make some changes to your diet and lifestyle if you have been diagnosed with non-alcoholic fatty liver disease. These diet and lifestyle changes include:

- Eating a lot of vegetables and fruits.
- Eating slow-release starchy foods, such as potatoes and bread.
- Doing regular exercises such as walking, jogging, or swimming.
- Reducing or stopping the consumption of alcohol.
- Avoiding refined sugars and saturated fats commonly found in chocolate, cakes, and biscuits.

Maintaining a healthy weight for your age and build is also recommended. If you have diabetes, it is suggested to work with your doctor to keep your blood sugar levels under good control. Consult your doctor if you have issues with high blood cholesterol levels or if you are insulin resistant.

Chronic Viral Hepatitis

If you suffer from a long-term hepatitis infection caused by a virus such as hepatitis B or hepatitis C and lasts for more than six to seven months, the condition is called Chronic Viral Hepatitis. In such a condition, it is recommended to eat a normal well-balanced diet. Fasting due for any reason is not recommended at all if you have chronic liver disease.

Maintaining an appropriate weight as per your height and build is highly recommended because it has been found in studies that more weight can increase and speed up the damages caused by hepatitis C and slow down the recovery.

Some studies show that some people have conditions like poor appetite, nausea, vomiting, and unintentional weight loss during treatment with anti-viral agents. If all or any of these conditions last for more than a few days, you must consult a doctor immediately.

Autoimmune Hepatitis

Autoimmune hepatitis is also categorized as chronic liver disease. It involves liver damage and inflammation due to an attack on the normal components and cells by the immune system. In a condition like this, sometimes, patients have prescribed steroids. In some cases, patients who have been prescribed steroids find that their appetite increases over time, and they gradually start gaining weight.

If you are suffering from autoimmune hepatitis and are on steroids and have symptoms like an increase in appetite and weight gain, it is still important and recommended to eat a well-balanced diet. If you are on steroids for a long time, you must be prescribed vitamin D and calcium by your doctor.

If, however, you start gaining more weight and it does not seem to slow down, you should try to reduce foods high in calories, such as:

- Sugar
- Cakes
- Fried food
- Pies and crisps
- Biscuits
- Chocolate
- Sweets
- Pasties

It is also recommended that you use low-fat milk and spreads and eat more fruit and vegetables. If it still increases, you must consult your doctor or dietician immediately

Chapter 2

Guidelines for a Forever Healthy Liver

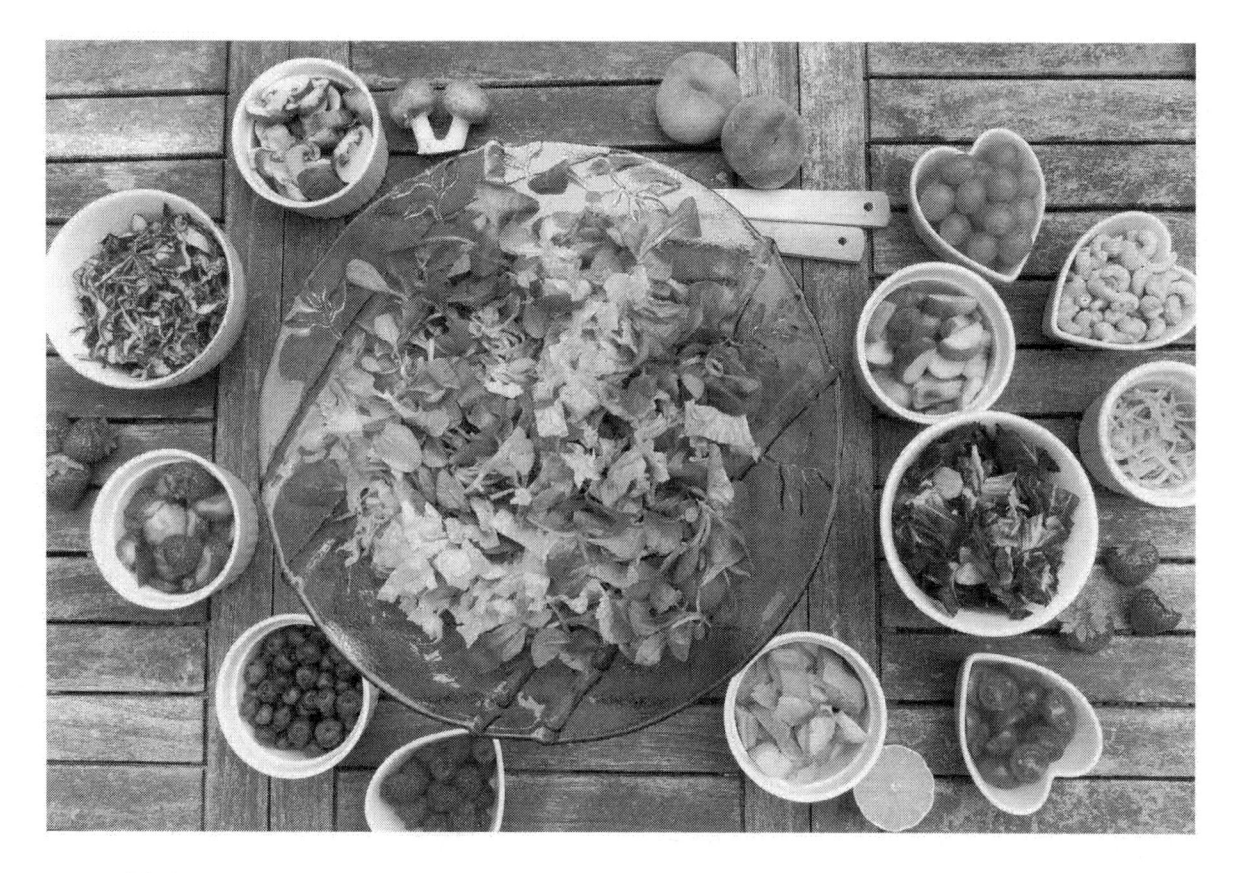

Eating a well-balanced diet is the easiest way to reverse and treat fatty liver disease.

- Remove or reduce from your diet fatty foods and foods that have a high level of sugar such as duck, pork belly, fried chips, crisps, nuts, etc.
- Eat lots of veggies.
- Avoid red meat.

- Avoid processed foods like lasagna, pizza, etc.; most of them are high in fat.
- Eat lean proteins such as fish, turkey, chicken, soy, and whole grains.
- Eliminate sodas, juices, and any sweet drinks.
- Substitute high-fat margarine, butter, lard, dripping, and mayonnaise with low-fat alternatives.
- Substitute full cream milk with skimmed or semi-skimmed milk.

You can reverse fatty liver automatically when the necessary steps are taken to treat obesity, an unhealthy diet, diabetes, and high cholesterol.

- Exercise regularly; it helps you get rid of excess liver fat—small workouts, brisk walking, etc.
- Stop drinking alcohol. This might not be easy for some people, but it's something you need to work on for your overall health benefit.
- Reduce carbs and sugar intake
- Be kind to your liver, and be mindful of your medications, especially those that can cause fatty liver.

Foods to Eat and Avoid

Food Group	Favorable for fatty liver	Rather unfavorable for fatty liver	In smaller quantities, mostly unproblematic
Vegetables	All vegetables, with the exceptions mentioned	Corn, sweet potatoes	
Fruit	Low-fructose fruits such as apples, berries, citrus fruits, papaya, watermelon, plums, nectarine, peach, apricot, avocado	Sugared fruit glasses and canned fruit, candied fruit	Bananas, grapes, sweet cherries, mango, honeydew melon
Grains, pulses, and starch suppliers	Filling cereals with a high protein content such as oatmeal, quinoa, amaranth, and all legumes	Bread and rolls made from extracted flour, white rice, milk rolls, sweet bits, and ready meals such as mashed potatoes, potato pancakes, or French fries	Products made from wholegrain flour, wholegrain rice, potatoes
Dairy products and eggs	Eggs, milk, and milk products with a fat content of up to 1.5%, cheeses with a fat content of up to 45%	Fatty dairy products such as cream, sour cream, crème fraîche, mayonnaise, sweetened finished products	
Meat and fish	Poultry, lean cold cuts such as salmon and boiled ham, turkey breast, sausage in aspic, all types of fish	Fatty sausages such as liver sausage, mortadella, bacon, meat loaf; fish, or meat breaded or pickled in fatty sauces	Fillet of beef and pork
Oils and fats	Vegetable oils such as linseed oil, nut oils, rapeseed oil, wheat germ oil, olive oil	Lard, palm fat, safflower and sunflower oil, butter	
Nuts and seeds	All types of nuts except the one mentioned	Ready-to-use nut mixes and salted nuts	Unsalted peanuts

Health Benefits of Various Foods

You need to know about the benefits of certain foods so that you might be able to incorporate them into your daily diet.

Cruciferous Vegetables

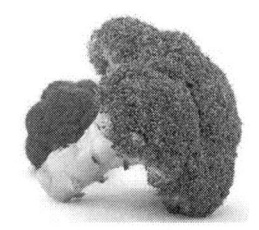

These vegetables have a high level of mineral sulfur, enhancing liver detoxification. Cruciferous vegetables include Brussels sprouts, broccoli, cabbage, broccolini, and cauliflower.

Leafy Greens

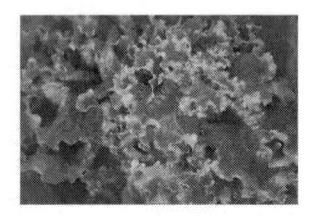

Dark, leafy green vegetables have high levels of chlorophyll and vitamin K, both extremely important for general health. Leafy green vegetables include bok choy, mustard greens, spinach, watercress, silverbeet, choy sum, and other Asian greens.

Bitter Greens

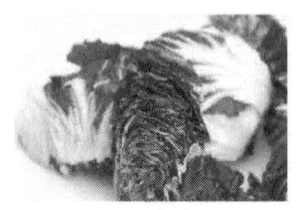

Bitter greens such as endive, radicchio, rocket, and chicory enhance bile flow.

Yogurt

Yogurt consists of certain friendly bacteria. Be sure to use plain, full-fat yogurt with no sweetener, or try Greek-style yogurt.

Omega-3 Fatty Acid-Rich Foods

Omega-3 fatty acids are required for the maintenance of healthy cell membranes. They can also be used to decrease the inflammation of the liver cells often seen in the fatty liver. Omega-3 fatty acids can be found in sardines, salmon, tuna, mackerel, trout, hemp, flaxseeds, chia seeds, walnuts, and grass-fed lambs.

Foods with Vitamin C

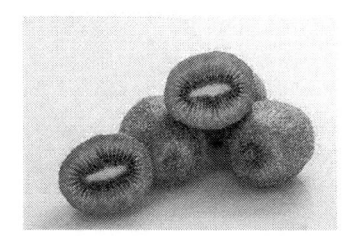

Vitamin C improves the function of the liver. The best sources for getting this vitamin are limes, lemons, oranges, grapefruits, kiwi fruit, mandarins, berries, tomatoes, and capsicums.

Onions and Garlic

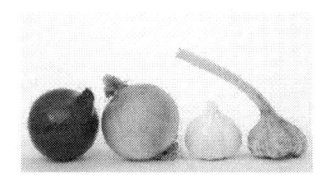

Both onion and garlic consist of certain cleansing products that purify the liver and blood. It should ideally be eaten regularly. The raw form is preferable but can be used in the cooked form.

Hummus and Tahini

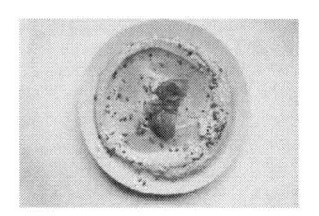

Tahini and hummus are both rich sources of minerals, calcium in particular. They also have high amounts of healthy fats.

Olives

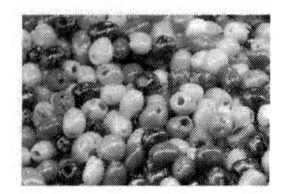

Both forms of olives, i.e., green and black, contain antioxidants and healthy fats.

Eggs

Eggs have a good amount of sulfur and protein. They are healthy for the liver and will not affect cholesterol levels. Eggs are useful if you are trying to lose weight and reverse fatty liver.

Avocados

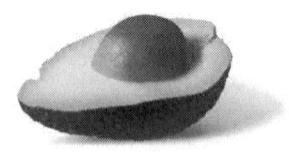

Avocados have high levels of vitamin E as compared to other food items. They are extremely healthy for liver health.

CHAPTER 3
BREAKFAST

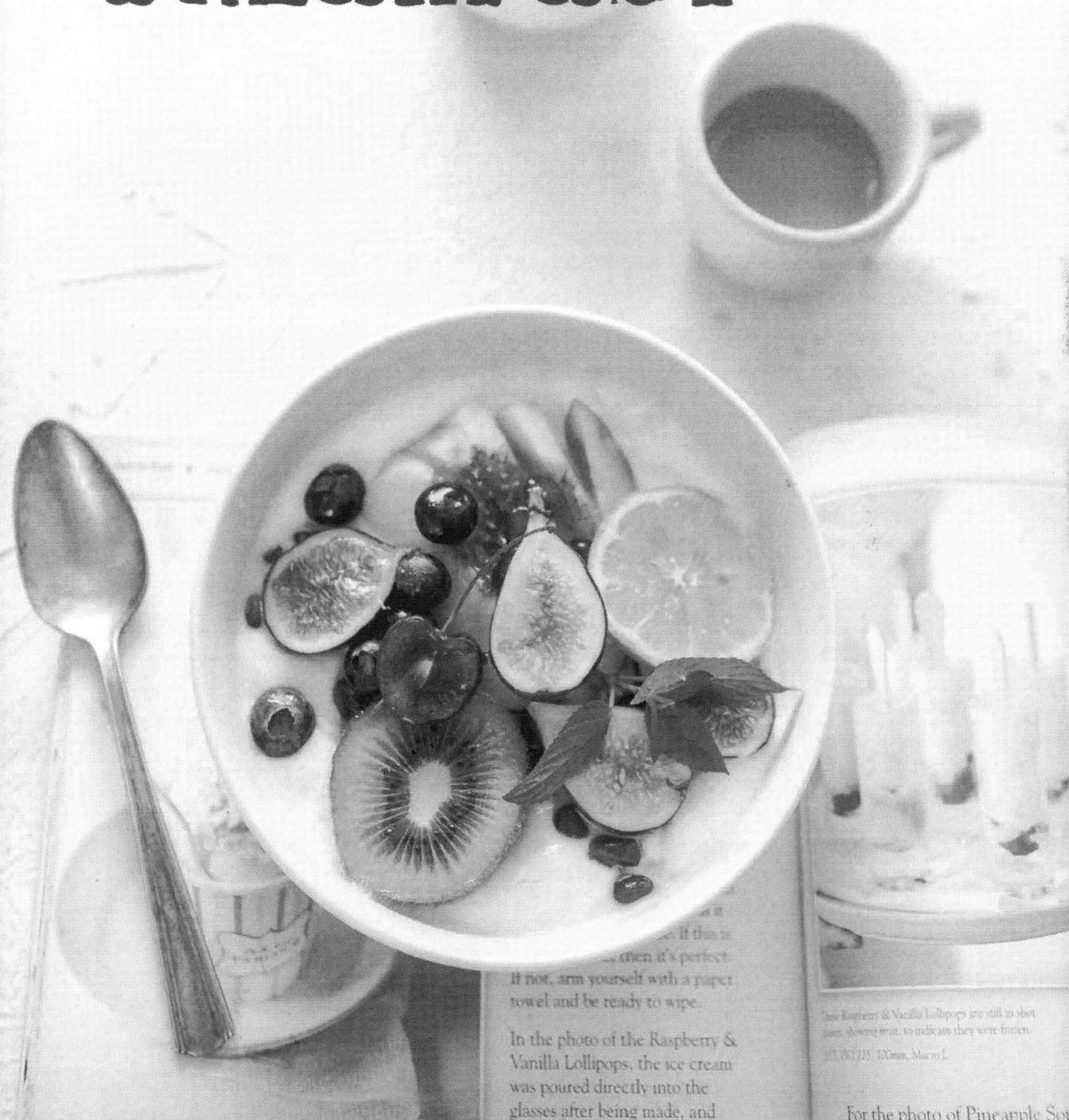

Cherry Berry Bulgur Bowl

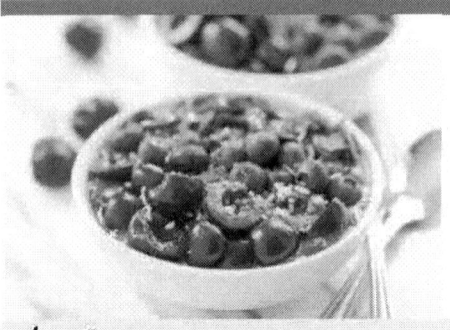

Preparation: 10 min
Cooking: 10 min
Servings: 4

Directions:

1. Mix the bulgur, water, and salt in a medium saucepan at medium heat. Bring to a boil.
2. Reduce the heat to low and simmer, partially covered, for 12 to 15 minutes or until the bulgur is almost tender. Cover, and let stand for 5 minutes to finish cooking after removing the pan from the heat.
3. While the bulgur is cooking, combine the raspberries and blackberries in a medium bowl. Stir the cherry jam into the fruit.
4. When the bulgur is tender, divide it among four bowls. Top each bowl with ½ cup of yogurt and an equal amount of the berry mixture, and serve.

Nutrition: Calories: 242 | Fats: 3 g | Carbs: 22 g | Protein: 9 g

Ingredients:

- 1 cup medium-grind bulgur
- 2 cups water
- Pinch salt
- 1 cup halved and pitted cherries or 1 cup canned cherries, drained
- ½ cup raspberries
- ½ cup blackberries
- 1 tablespoon cherry jam
- 2 cups plain whole-milk yogurt

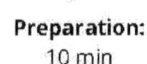

Baked Curried Apple Oatmeal Cups

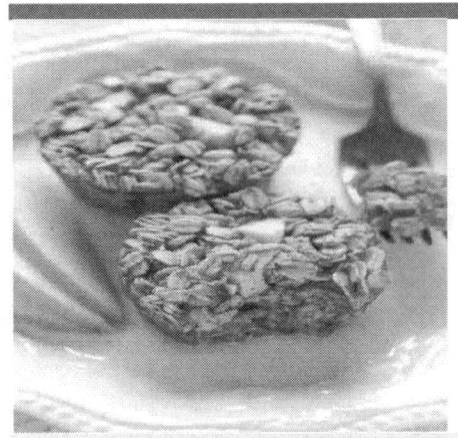

Preparation: 10 min
Cooking: 10 min
Servings: 4

Directions:

1. Preheat the oven to 375°F. Then coat a 12-cup muffin tin with baking spray and set aside.
5. Combine the oats, brown sugar, curry powder, and salt in a medium bowl.
6. Mix the milk, applesauce, and vanilla in a small bowl,
7. Stir the liquid ingredients into the dry ingredients and mix until just combined. Stir in the walnuts.
8. Divide the mixture among the muffin cups using a scant ⅓ cup for each.
9. Bake this for 18 to 20 minutes until the oatmeal is firm. Serve.

Nutrition: Calories: 296 | Fats: 10 g | Sat Carbs: 45 g | Protein: 8 g

Ingredients:

- 3 ½ cups old-fashioned oats
- 3 tablespoons brown sugar
- 2 teaspoons preferred curry powder
- ⅛ teaspoon salt
- 1 cup unsweetened almond milk
- 1 cup unsweetened applesauce
- 1 teaspoon vanilla
- ½ cup chopped walnuts

Healthy Millet Porridge

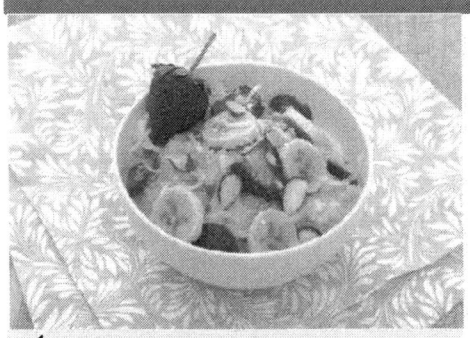

Preparation: 10 min | **Cooking:** 30 min | **Servings:** 2

Directions:

1. Grind millet in a food processor; set aside.
2. Toast almonds and walnuts in a nonstick skillet over medium-high heat for about 5 minutes or until golden brown. Stir in coconut and almonds, toast for 5 minutes more, and then remove from heat.
3. Add millet to the skillet and toast for about 3 minutes or until fragrant. Stir in 1 ½ cups of almond milk and bring to a gentle boil; lower the heat and simmer for about 10 minutes. Stir in half of the toasted coconut and almonds, cinnamon, and nutmeg and simmer for another 10 minutes.
4. Serve the porridge in two bowls and top with the remaining almond milk and toasted seed mixture.

Nutrition: Calories: 397 | Total Fats: 14.6 g | Total Carbs: 31.7 g | Protein: 12.6 g

Ingredients:

- 2 cups unsweetened almond milk
- ½ cup hulled millet
- 2 tablespoons slivered almonds
- 2 tablespoons shredded unsweetened coconut
- ¼ teaspoon ground nutmeg
- ½ teaspoon ground cinnamon

Peanut Butter and Cacao Breakfast Quinoa

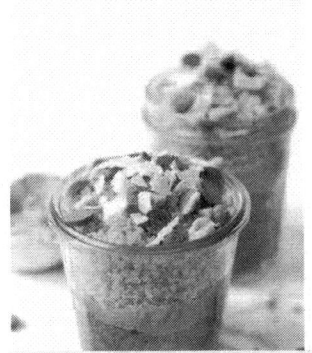

Preparation: 5 min | **Cooking:** 10 min | **Servings:** 1

Directions:

1. Using an 8-quart pot over medium-high heat, stir together the quinoa flakes, milk, water, cacao powder, peanut butter, and cinnamon. Cook and stir until the mixture begins to simmer. Turn the heat to medium-low and cook for 3 to 5 minutes, stirring frequently.
2. Stir in the bananas and cook until hot.
3. Serve topped with fresh berries, nuts, and a splash of milk.

Nutrition: Calories: 471 | Fats: 16 g | Protein: 18 g | Carbs: 69 g |

Ingredients:

- 1/3 cup quinoa flakes
- ½ cup unsweetened nondairy milk
- ½ cup water
- 1/8 cup raw cacao powder
- 1 tablespoon natural creamy peanut butter
- 1/8 teaspoon ground cinnamon
- 1 banana, mashed
- Fresh berries of choice, for serving
- Chopped nuts of choice, for serving

Egg and Veggie Muffins

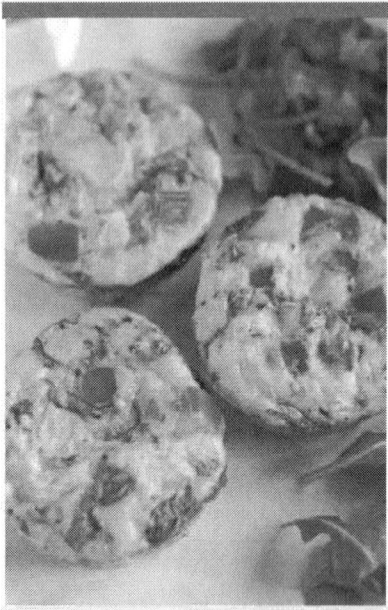

Preparation: 15 min | **Cooking:** 20 min | **Servings:** 4

Directions:

1. Preheat the oven to 350°F.
2. Coat 4 muffin pans with cooking spray. Set aside.
3. Whisk together the milk, eggs, onion, red pepper, parsley, red pepper flakes, and black pepper until mixed.
4. Pour the egg mixture into prepared muffin pans.
5. Bake until the muffins are puffed and golden, about 18 to 20 minutes.
6. Serve

Nutrition: Calories: 84 | Fats: 5 g | Carbs: 3 g | Protein: 7 g

Ingredients:

- Cooking spray
- 4 eggs
- 2 tablespoons unsweetened rice milk
- ½ sweet onion, chopped
- ½ red bell pepper, chopped
- Pinch red pepper flakes
- Pinch ground black pepper

Breakfast Tacos

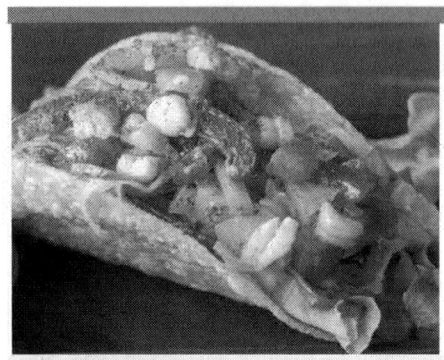

Preparation: 10 min | **Cooking:** 10 min | **Servings:** 4

Directions:

1. Heat the oil in a large skillet at medium flame.
2. Add the onion, bell pepper, and garlic; sauté until softened, about 5 minutes.
3. Add the eggs, cumin, and red pepper flakes. Scramble the eggs with the vegetables until cooked through and fluffy.
4. Spoon one-fourth of the egg mixture into the center of each tortilla, and top each with 1 tablespoon of salsa.
5. Serve immediately.

Nutrition: Calories: 211 | Total Fats: 7 g | Carbs: 17 g | Protein: 9 g

Ingredients:

- 1 teaspoon olive oil
- ½ sweet onion, chopped
- ½ red bell pepper, chopped
- ½ teaspoon minced garlic
- 4 eggs, beaten
- ½ teaspoon ground cumin
- Pinch red pepper flakes
- 4 tortillas
- ¼ cup tomato salsa

Vegetable Omelet

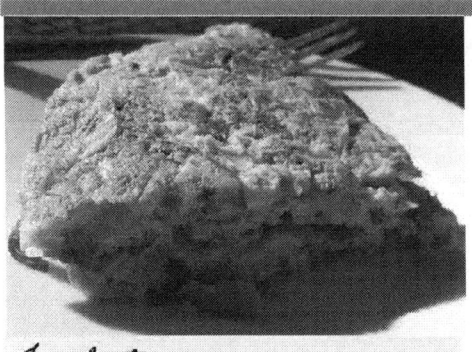

Preparation: 15 min | **Cooking:** 10 min | **Servings:** 3

Ingredients:
- 4 egg whites
- 1 egg
- 2 tablespoons chopped fresh parsley
- 2 tablespoons water
- Olive oil spray
- ½ cup chopped and boiled red bell pepper
- ¼ cup chopped scallion, both green and white parts
- Ground black pepper

Directions:
1. Whisk together the egg, egg whites, parsley, and water until well blended. Set aside.
2. Spray a skillet with olive oil spray and heat over medium flame.
3. Sauté the peppers and scallion for 3 minutes or until softened.
4. Over the vegetables, you can now pour the egg and cook, swirling the skillet, for 2 minutes or until the edges start to set. Cook until set.
5. Season with black pepper and serve.

Nutrition: Calories: 77 | Fats: 3 g | Carbs: 2 g | Protein: 12 g

Buckwheat and Grapefruit Porridge

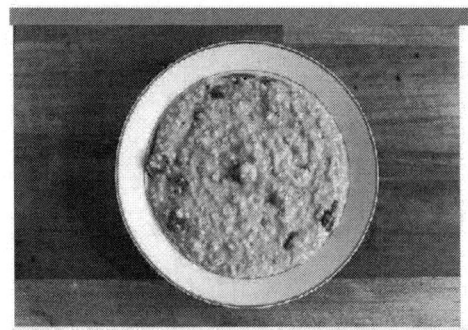

Preparation: 5 min | **Cooking:** 20 min | **Servings:** 2

Ingredients:
- ½ cup buckwheat
- ¼ grapefruit, chopped
- 1 tablespoon honey
- 1 ½ cups almond milk
- 2 cups water

Directions:
1. Boil water on the stove. Add the buckwheat and place the lid on the pan.
2. Simmer for 7 to 10 minutes in low heat. Check to ensure the water does not dry out.
3. Remove and set aside for 5 minutes, do this when most of the water is absorbed.
4. Drain excess water from the pan and stir in almond milk, heating through for 5 minutes.
5. Add the honey and grapefruit.
6. Serve.

Nutrition: Calories: 231 | Fats: 4 g | Carbs: 43 g

Raspberry Pudding

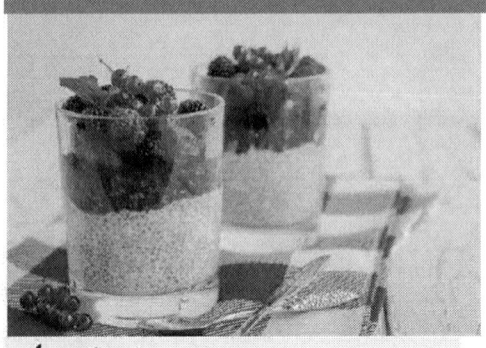

Preparation: 10 min
Cooking: 30 min
Servings: 2

Directions:

1. Mix plain yogurt with maple syrup and ground cardamom.
2. Add chia seeds. Stir it gently.
3. Put the yogurt in the serving glasses and top with the raspberries.
4. Refrigerate the breakfast for at least 30 minutes or overnight.

Nutrition: Calories: 303 | Fats: 11.2 g | Carbs: 33.2 g| Protein: 15.5 g

Ingredients:

- ½ cup raspberries
- 2 teaspoons maple syrup
- 1 ½ cup plain yogurt
- ¼ teaspoon ground cardamom
- 1/3 cup chia seeds, dried

Pineapple, Macha & Beet Chia Pudding

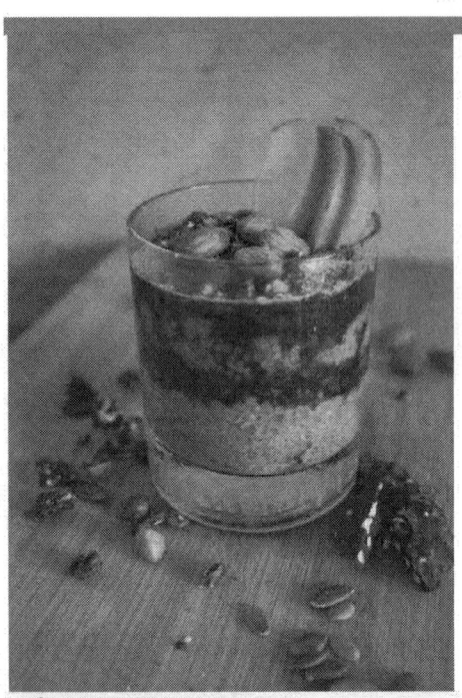

Preparation: 10 min
Cooking: 0 min
Servings: 4

Directions:

Green Chia pudding layer:

1. Add half each of chia seeds, raw honey, almond milk, and matcha green tea powder to the blender and until very smooth, transfer to a bowl.

Beetroot layer:

1. Combine beetroot and ginger with the remaining chia seeds, raw honey, vanilla, and coconut milk until smooth; transfer to a separate bowl. In a food processor, puree the fresh pineapple until fine.
2. To assemble, layer the chia pudding in the bottom of serving glasses, followed by the pureed pineapple and then the beetroot layer. Top with figs and toasted almonds for a crunchy finish.

Nutrition: Calories: 421 | Fats: 23.5 g | Carbs: 22.3 g| Protein: 1.8 g

Ingredients:

- 1 cup chia seeds
- 1 teaspoon raw honey
- 2 cups almond milk
- 1 teaspoon matcha green tea powder
- 2 tablespoons fresh beetroot juice
- 1 whole pineapple
- 1 cup freshly squeezed lemon juice
- 1 knob fresh ginger
- Toasted almonds and figs to serve

Tapioca Pudding

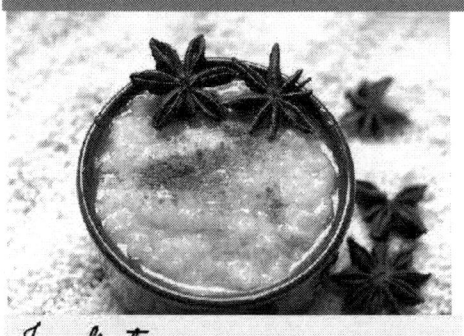

Preparation: 10 min
Cooking: 15 min
Servings: 3

Ingredients:
- ¼ cup pearl tapioca
- ¼ cup maple syrup
- 2 cups almond milk
- ½ cup coconut flesh, shredded
- 1 and ½ teaspoon lemon juice

Directions:
1. In a pan, combine milk with tapioca and the rest of the ingredients, bring to a simmer over medium heat, and cook for 15 minutes.
2. Divide the mix into bowls, cool it down, and serve for breakfast.

Nutrition: Calories: 361 | Fats: 28.5 g | Carbs: 28.3 g | Protein: 2.8 g

Banana Pancakes

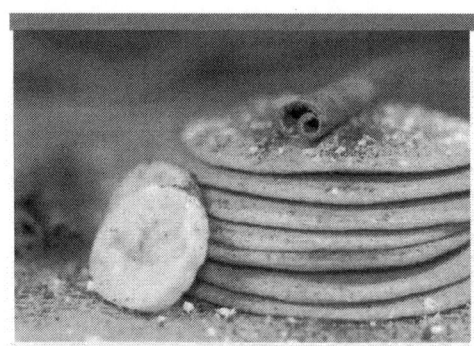

Preparation: 10 min
Cooking: 20 min
Servings: 4

Ingredients:
- 1 cup whole wheat flour
- ¼ teaspoon baking soda
- ¼ teaspoon baking powder
- 1 cup mashed banana
- 2 eggs
- 1 cup skim milk

Directions:
1. In a bowl, combine all ingredients and mix well.
2. In a skillet, heat olive oil.
3. Pour ¼ of the batter and cook each pancake for 1-2 minutes per side.
4. When ready, remove from heat and serve.

Nutrition: Calories: 210 | Carbs: 8 g | Fats: 13 g | Protein: 15 g

Nectarine Pancakes

Ingredients:
- 1 cup whole wheat flour
- ¼ teaspoon baking soda
- ¼ teaspoon baking powder
- 1 cup nectarines
- 2 eggs
- 1 cup skim milk

Preparation: 10 min

Cooking: 30 min

Servings: 4

Directions:
1. In a bowl, combine all ingredients and mix well.
2. In a skillet, heat olive oil.
3. Pour ¼ of the batter and cook each pancake for 1-2 minutes per side.
4. When ready, remove from heat and serve.

Nutrition: Calories: 210 | Carbs: 7 g | Fats: 14 g | Protein: 15 g

Pancakes

Ingredients:
- 1 cup whole wheat flour
- ¼ teaspoon baking soda
- ¼ teaspoon baking powder
- 2 eggs
- 1 cup skim milk

Preparation: 10 min

Cooking: 30 min

Servings: 4

Directions:
1. In a bowl, combine all ingredients and mix well.
2. In a skillet, heat olive oil.
3. Pour ¼ of the batter and cook each pancake for 1-2 minutes per side.
4. When ready, remove from heat and serve.

Nutrition: Calories: 100 | Carbs: 2 g | Fat: 6 g | Protein: 10 g

Peach Muffins

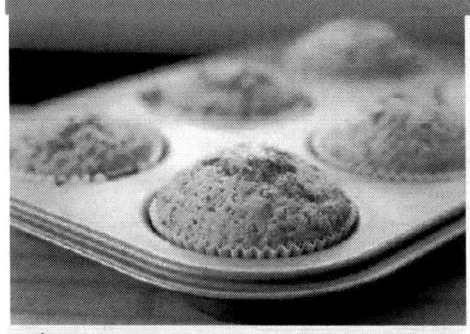

Preparation: 10 min

Cooking: 30 min

Servings: 4

Ingredients:

- 2 eggs
- 1 tablespoon olive oil
- 1 cup skim milk
- 2 cups whole wheat flour
- 1 teaspoon baking soda
- ¼ teaspoon baking soda
- 1 cup peaches
- 1 teaspoon cinnamon
- ¼ cup molasses

Directions:

1. In a bowl, combine all wet ingredients.
2. In another bowl, combine all dry ingredients.
3. Combine wet and dry ingredients.
4. Pour the mixture into 8-12 preparation muffin cups; fill 2/3 of the cups.
5. Bake for 18-20 minutes at 375°F.
6. When ready, remove and serve.

Nutrition: Calories 100 | Carbs: 2 g | Fats: 5 g | Protein: 10 g

Blueberry Muffins

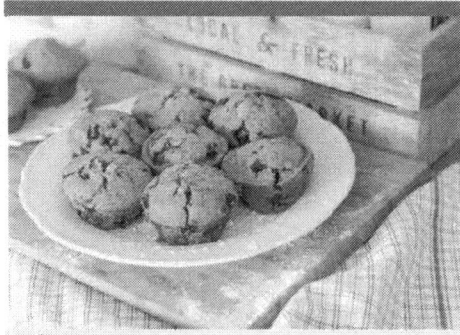

Preparation: 10 min

Cooking: 30 min

Servings: 4

Ingredients:

- 2 eggs
- 1 tablespoon olive oil
- 1 cup skim milk
- 2 cups whole wheat flour
- 1 teaspoon baking soda
- ¼ teaspoon baking soda
- 1 teaspoon cinnamon
- 1 cup blueberries

Directions:

1. In a bowl, combine all wet ingredients.
2. In another bowl, combine all dry ingredients.
3. Combine wet and dry ingredients.
4. Fold in blueberries and mix well.
5. Pour the mixture into 8-12 preparation muffin cups; fill 2/3 of the cups.
6. Bake for 18-20 minutes at 375°F.
7. When ready, remove and serve.

Nutrition: Calories 100 | Carbs: 2 g | Fats: 5 g | Protein: 10 g

Avocado Spread

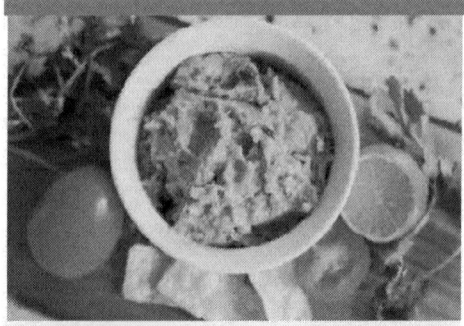

Preparation: 10 min | **Cooking:** 0 min | **Servings:** 8

Directions:
1. Put the avocados in a bowl and mash with a fork.
2. Add the rest of the ingredients, stir to combine, and serve as a morning spread.

Nutrition: Calories: 110 | Fats: 10 g | Carbs: 5.7 g | Protein: 1.2 g

Ingredients:
- 2 avocados, peeled, pitted, and roughly chopped
- 1 tablespoon sun-dried tomatoes, chopped
- 2 tablespoons lemon juice
- 3 tablespoons cherry tomatoes, chopped
- ¼ cup red onion, chopped
- 1 teaspoon oregano, dried
- 2 tablespoons parsley, chopped
- 4 kalamata olives, pitted and chopped
- A pinch salt and black pepper

Deviled eggs

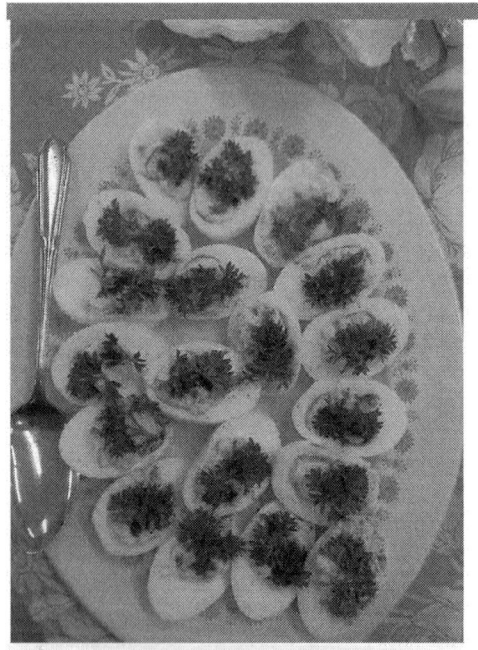

Preparation: 10 min | **Cooking:** 20 min | **Servings:** 8

Directions:
1. In a saucepan, add the eggs and bring to a boil.
2. Cover and boil for 10-15 minutes.
3. When ready, slice the eggs in half and remove the yolks.
4. In a bowl, combine the remaining ingredients and mix well.
5. Spoon 1 tablespoon of the mixture into each egg.
6. Garnish with green onions and serve.

Nutrition: Calories: 460 | Carbs: 35 g | Fats: 30 g | Protein: 20 g

Ingredients:
- 8 eggs
- ½ cup Greek yogurt
- 1 tablespoon mustard
- 1 teaspoon smoked paprika
- 1 tablespoon green onions

Spicy Cucumbers

Ingredients:
- 2 cucumbers
- 1 cup Greek yogurt
- 1 garlic clove
- 1 teaspoon paprika
- 1 teaspoon dill
- 1 teaspoon chili powder

Preparation: 10 min
Cooking: 20 min
Servings: 7

Directions:
1. In a bowl, combine all ingredients except cucumbers
2. Cut the cucumbers into rounds and scoot out the inside.
3. Fill each cucumber with the spicy mixture.
4. When ready, sprinkle paprika and serve.

Nutrition: Calories: 165 | Carbs: 3 g | Fats: 10 g | Protein : 12 g

Herbed Spinach Frittata

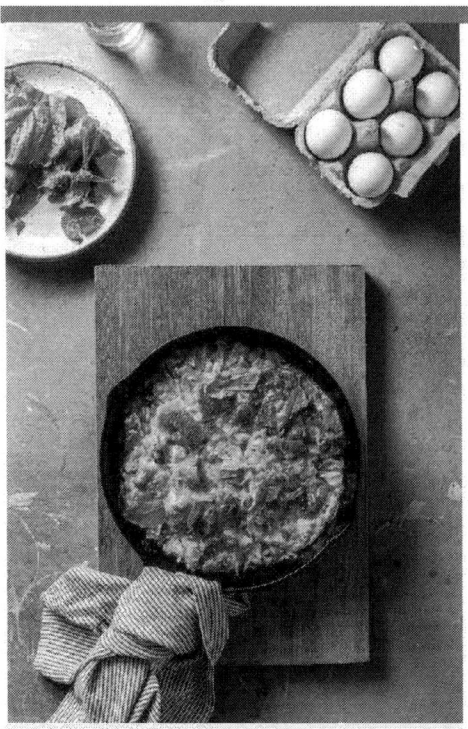

Ingredients:
- 5 eggs, beaten
- 1 cup fresh spinach
- 2 oz Parmesan, grated
- 1/3 cup cherry tomatoes
- ½ teaspoon dried oregano
- 1 teaspoon dried thyme
- 1 teaspoon olive oil

Preparation: 10 min
Cooking: 20 min
Servings: 4

Directions:
1. Chop the spinach into tiny pieces and or use a blender.
2. Then combine chopped spinach with eggs, dried oregano, and thyme.
3. Add Parmesan and stir the frittata mixture with the help of the fork.
4. Brush the springform pan with olive oil and pour the egg mixture inside.
5. Cut the cherry tomatoes into halves and place them over the egg mixture.
6. Preheat the oven to 360°F.
7. Bake the frittata for 20 minutes or until it is solid.
8. Chill the cooked breakfast till the room temperature and slice into the servings.

Nutrition: Calories: 140 | Fats: 9.8 | Carbs: 2.1 | Protein: 11.9

Pumpkin Flax Granola

This recipe is crunchy and satisfying! Serve with smoothie or yogurt.

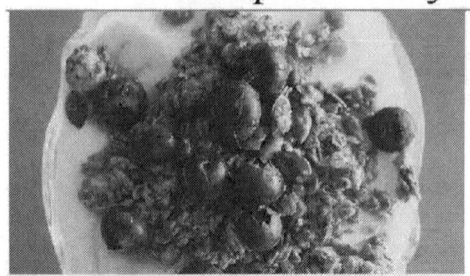

Preparation: 25 min | **Cooking:** 5 min | **Servings:** 19

Ingredients:
- 1 cup pumpkin seeds shelled
- 3 cups rolled oats old fashioned whole grain
- ¼ cup flax seeds
- ¼ cup honey
- ¼ cup maple syrup
- ½ cup sugar-free coconut flakes
- ¼ cup olive oil
- ½ teaspoons salt

Directions:
1. Preheat the oven to 325°F.
2. Combine the oats, pumpkin seeds, coconut flakes, and flax seeds in a large bowl.
3. Combine oil, maple syrup, honey, and salt in a microwave-safe bowl, stir well, and microwave for 30 seconds.
4. Slowly drizzle the liquid mixture into the dry mixture and stir gently until well coated.
5. Prepare a large baking sheet with parchment paper. Pour the mixture onto the baking sheet, place it in the heated oven, and bake for 20 minutes. Stir once in the middle of the time.
6. Remove from heat, set aside to cool down before crumbling with your hands, and then store in an airtight container at room temperature.
7. Serve with a smoothie or yogurt of choice, enjoy!

Nutrition: Calories: 113 | Protein: 2 g | Carbs: 13 g

Broiled Parmesan Avocado

This recipe is loaded with nutrients and is quick to put together.

Ingredients:
- 1 avocado, halved and pitted
- 2 tablespoons parmesan cheese grated
- 1 lime juice and zest
- Salt and pepper to taste

Preparation: 14 min | **Cooking:** 10 min | **Servings:** 4

Directions:
1. Heat the toaster oven to broil.
2. Squeeze lime, sprinkle parmesan cheese, lime zest, salt, and pepper to taste over avocado
3. Broil until cheese is melted, for about 4 minutes.
4. Remove from heat and serve immediately.

Nutrition: Calories: 61 | Protein: 4 g | Carbs: 4 g | Fats: 2 g |

Mexican Scrambled Eggs in Tortilla

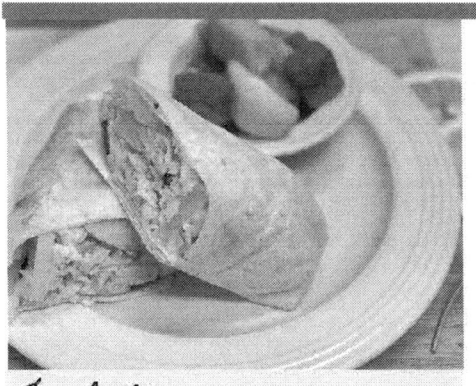

Preparation: 5 min | **Cooking:** 20 min | **Servings:** 2

Directions:

1. Coat a medium skillet with some cooking spray and heat for a few seconds.
2. Whisk the eggs with the green chilies, hot sauce, and cumin.
3. Add the eggs to the pan, and whisk with a spatula to scramble. Add the salt.
4. Cook until fluffy and done (1-2 minutes) over low heat.
5. Open the tortillas and spread 1 tablespoon of salsa on each.
6. Distribute the egg mixture onto the tortillas and wrap gently to make a burrito.
7. Serve warm.

Nutrition: Calories: 44.1 | Carbs: 2.23 g | Protein: 17.69 g | Fats: 0.39 g

Ingredients:

- 2 medium corn tortillas
- 4 egg whites
- 1 teaspoon cumin
- 3 teaspoons green chilies, diced
- ½ teaspoon hot pepper sauce
- 2 tablespoons salsa
- ½ teaspoon salt

Raspberry Overnight Porridge

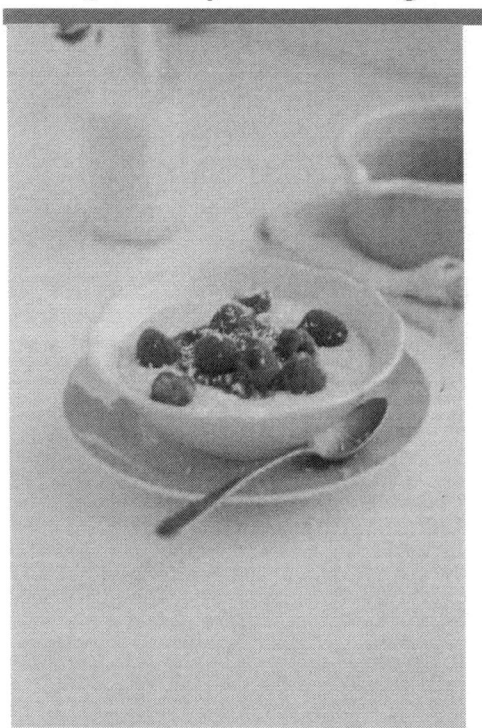

- 5-6 raspberries, fresh or canned and unsweetened

Preparation: overnight | **Cooking:** 0 min | **Servings:** 12

Directions:

1. Combine the oats, almond milk, and honey in a mason jar and place them in the fridge overnight.
2. Serve the next morning with the raspberries on top.

Nutrition: Calories: 143.6 | Carbs: 34.62 g | Protein: 3.44 g | Fats: 3.91 g

Ingredients:

- ⅓ cup rolled oats
- ½ cup almond milk
- 1 tablespoon honey

Turkey and Spinach Scramble on Melba Toast

Ingredients:
- 1 teaspoon extra virgin olive oil
- 1 cup raw spinach
- ½ garlic clove, minced
- 1 teaspoon nutmeg, grated
- 1 cup cooked and diced turkey breast
- 4 slices melba toast
- 1 teaspoon balsamic vinegar

Preparation: 2 min
Cooking: 15 min
Servings: 2

Directions:
1. Heat a pot and add oil.
2. Add turkey and heat through for 6 to 8 minutes.
3. Add spinach, garlic, and nutmeg and stir-fry for 6 minutes more.
4. Plate up the Melba toast and top with spinach and turkey scramble.
5. Drizzle with balsamic vinegar and serve.

Nutrition: Calories: 301 | Fats: 19 g | Carbs: 12 g | Protein: 19 g

Mexican Style Burritos

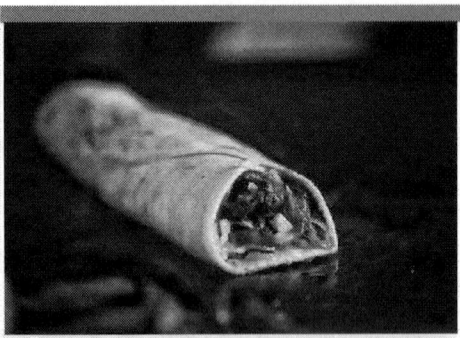

Preparation: 5 min
Cooking: 15 min
Servings: 2

Directions:
1. Turn the broiler to medium heat and place the tortillas underneath for 1 to 2 minutes on each side or until lightly toasted.
2. Remove and keep the broiler on.
3. Sauté onion, chili, and bell peppers for 5 to 6 minutes or until soft.
4. Place the eggs on top of the onions and peppers and place the skillet under the broiler for 5-6 minutes or until the eggs are cooked.
5. Serve half the eggs and vegetables on top of each tortilla and sprinkle with cilantro and lime juice to serve.

Nutrition: Calories: 202 | Fats: 13 g | Carbs: 19 g | Protein: 9 g

Ingredients:
- 1 tablespoon olive oil
- 2 corn tortillas
- ¼ cup red onion, chopped
- ¼ cup red bell peppers, chopped
- ½ red chili, deseeded and chopped
- 2 eggs
- Juice of 1 lime
- 1 tablespoon cilantro, chopped

Quinoa Bowls With Avocado and Egg

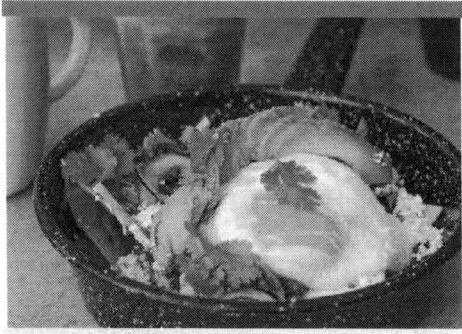

Preparation: 10 min

Cooking: 25 min

Servings: 5

Ingredients:

- 5 hard-boiled eggs, peeled and sliced
- 3 avocados, pitted, sliced, and coated with lemon juice
- 3¾ cups cooked quinoa
- ½ teaspoon onion powder
- ½ teaspoon freshly ground black pepper
- ½ teaspoon ground cumin
- ½ teaspoon garlic powder
- 1 tablespoon chopped fresh cilantro
- 2 small tomatoes, diced
- ½ large red onion, chopped

Directions:

1. In a large bowl, season the cooked quinoa with the onion powder, pepper, cumin, and garlic powder. Add the cilantro, tomatoes, and onion and mix well.
2. Divide the quinoa mix among 5 storage containers as a base for the breakfast bowl; then divide the avocados evenly into the bowls. Top each with a whole sliced egg.
3. Storage: Seal airtight, and store in the refrigerator for up to 5 days. This dish may be served cold or warm. If warm is preferred, separate the egg and avocado from the quinoa mixture. Reheat the quinoa in the microwave for 1 minute. Then top with the egg and avocado.

Nutrition: Calories: 388 | Total Fats: 20 g | Carbs: 40 g | Protein: 15 g

Chapter 4

VEGETARIAN MAINS

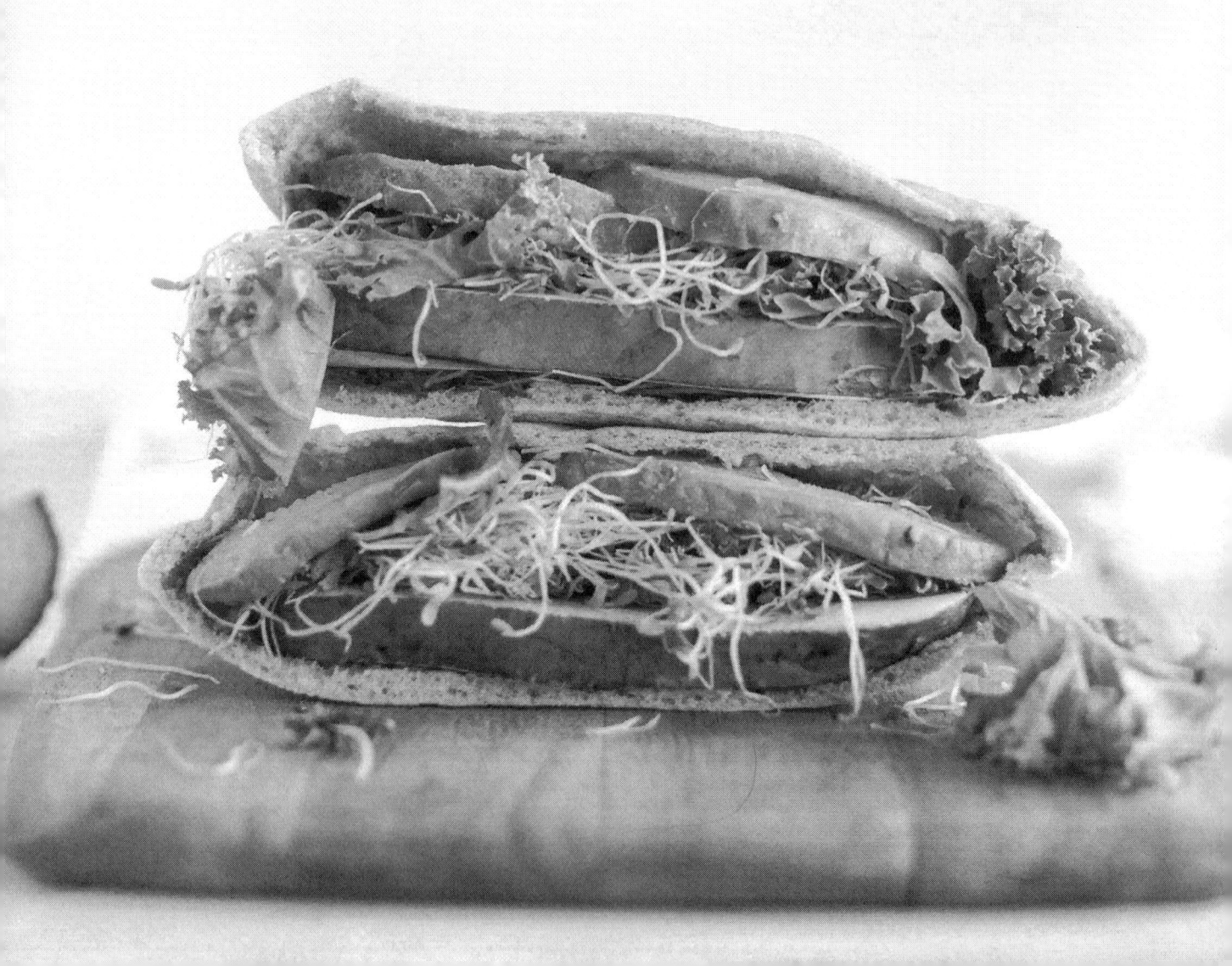

Tofu Rice

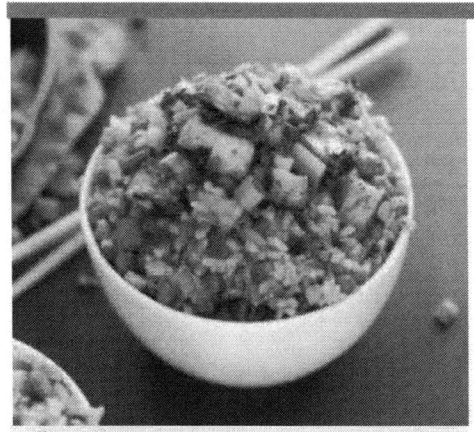

Preparation: 10 min | **Cooking:** 13 min | **Servings:** 4

Directions:
1. Sauce tofu with peas, carrots, garlic powder, soy sauce, scallions, black pepper, and salt in a cooking pan for 10 minutes.
2. Stir in cauliflower rice and mix well.
3. Cover and cook for 3 minutes on medium heat.
4. Serve warm.

Serving Suggestion: Serve the rice with kale salad.
Variation tip: Add boiled couscous to the mixture.
Nutrition: Calories: 378 | Fats: 3.8 g | Carbs: 13.3 g | Protein: 5.4 g

Ingredients:
- 1 package baked tofu
- 4 cup cauliflower rice
- 1 cup frozen peas
- 1 cup carrots, shredded
- 1 teaspoon onion powder
- 1 teaspoon garlic powder
- ½ cup soy sauce
- ¼ cup scallions, chopped
- Salt and black pepper to taste

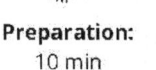

Green Buddha Bowl

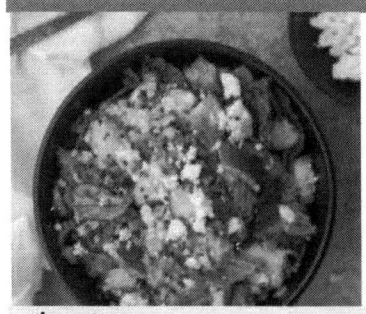

Preparation: 15 min | **Cooking:** 0 min | **Servings:** 2

Directions:
1. Mix quinoa with apple and the rest of the ingredients in a salad bowl.
2. Serve.

Serving Suggestion: Serve the bowl with spaghetti squash.
Variation tip: Add some edamame beans to the bowl.
Nutrition: Calories: 318 | Fats: 15.7 g | Carbs: 27 g | Protein: 4.9 g

Ingredients:
- 1 tablespoon olive oil
- 1 lb. brussels sprouts, trimmed and halved
- Salt and black pepper to taste
- 2 cups cooked quinoa
- 1 cup red apple, chopped
- ¼ cup pepitas
- 1 avocado, sliced
- 1 ½ cups arugula
- ½ cup mayo
- ¾ cup plain Greek yogurt
- 1 teaspoon ground mustard
- ¼ cup Pompeian white balsamic vinegar
- 1 tablespoon fresh basil, chopped
- 1 garlic clove, minced

Tofu Spinach Sauté

Ingredients:
- ¼ cup onion, chopped
- ¼ cup button mushrooms, chopped
- 8 ounces tofu, pressed and chopped
- 3 teaspoons nutritional yeast
- 1 teaspoon liquid aminos
- 4 cups baby spinach
- 4 grape tomatoes, chopped
- Cooking spray

Preparation: 10 min
Cooking: 10 min
Servings: 4

Directions:
1. Sauté mushrooms and onion with oil in a skillet for 3 minutes.
2. Stir in tofu and sauté for 3 minutes.
3. Add liquid aminos and yeast, then mix well.
4. Stir in tomatoes and spinach, then sauté for 4 minutes.
5. Serve warm.

Serving Suggestion: Serve the tofu with kale salad.
Variation tip: Add boiled couscous to the mixture.
Nutrition: Calories: 378 | Fats: 3.8 g | Carbs: 13.3 g | Protein: 5.4 g

Roasted Green Beans and Mushrooms

Ingredients:
- 8 ounces mushrooms, cleaned and halved
- 1 lb. green beans, halved
- 8 whole garlic cloves, halved
- 2 tablespoons olive oil
- 1 tablespoon balsamic vinegar
- Salt and black pepper to taste

Preparation: 15 min
Cooking: 25 min
Servings: 4

Directions:
1. At 450°F, preheat your oven.
2. Spread a foil sheet on a baking tray.
3. Add mushrooms, garlic, and green beans to the baking sheet.
4. Mix balsamic vinegar with olive oil in a small bowl and pour over the veggies.
5. Drizzle black pepper and salt on top, then bake for 25 minutes.
6. Serve warm.

Serving Suggestion: Serve the veggies with toasted bread slices.
Variation tip: Add boiled zucchini pasta to the mixture.
Nutrition: Calories: 136 | Fats: 6 g | Carbs: 8 g | Fiber: 2 g | Protein: 4 g

Vegetable and Egg Casserole

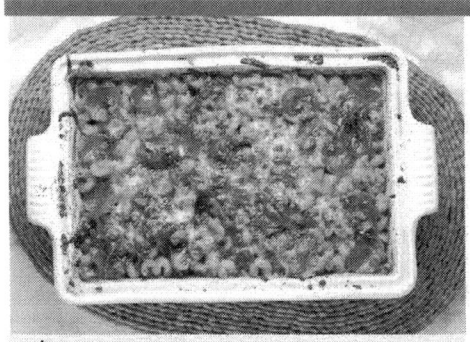

Preparation: 15 min
Cooking: 30 min
Servings: 6

Directions:

1. At 350°F, preheat your oven.
2. Beat egg with egg whites, cheese, spinach, tomatoes, mushrooms, and bell pepper in a bowl.
3. Spread this egg mixture into a casserole dish.
4. Bake this casserole for 30 minutes in the oven.
5. Serve warm.

Serving Suggestion: Serve the casserole with cauliflower salad.
Variation tip: Top the casserole with onion slices before cooking.
Nutrition: Calories: 341 | Fats: 24 g | Carbs 36.4 g | Protein: 10.3 g

Ingredients:

- 6 eggs
- 1 cup egg whites
- 1 ¼ cup cheese, shredded
- 16 ounces bag frozen spinach
- 2 cups mushrooms, sliced
- 1 bell pepper, diced
- 10 cherry tomatoes, sliced

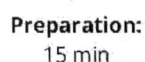

Zucchini Boat

Ingredients:

- 2 medium zucchinis
- 2 tablespoons olive oil
- ½ medium onion, diced
- 2 garlic cloves, minced
- 1 can corn, drained
- 1 cup enchilada sauce
- ½ teaspoons salt or to taste
- ½ cup white mushrooms
- ½ cup bok choy, chopped
- 1 teaspoon cumin
- ½ cup parmesan cheese

Preparation: 25 min
Cooking: 20 min
Servings: 2

Directions:

1. Wash and cut the zucchini lengthwise.
2. Heat oil in a skillet and sauté onions.
3. Then add garlic cloves and cook. Add in vegetables and cook until tender.
4. Add salt, enchilada sauce, and cumin, and mix well.
5. Turn off the heat and let it get cool.
6. Scoop out the seeds of the zucchini.
7. Fill the cavity of zucchini with a bowl mixture.
8. Top it with a handful of Parmesan cheese.
9. Arrange four zucchinis in the Air Fryer basket.
10. Select the Air Fry mode for 20 minutes and adjust the temperature to 390°F.
11. Once done, serve and enjoy.

Serving Suggestion: Serve it with ketchup
Variation tip: None
Nutrition: Calories:472 | Fats: 28.2 g | Carbs: 40.5 g | Protein: 26.5 g

Zucchini Cups

Ingredients:
- 4 cup grated zucchini
- 2 large eggs
- ½ cup parmesan cheese
- 2 teaspoons almond flour.
- 1 teaspoon sesame seeds
- Salt, to taste

Preparation: 10 min
Cooking: 8 min
Servings: 4

Directions:
1. Preheat the Air Fryer to 400°F for 10 minutes.
2. First, wash and grate the zucchini and add salt.
3. Let it sit for 20 minutes.
4. Squeeze it to drain excess zucchini.
5. Add zucchini to the bowl and add eggs, parmesan cheese, sesame seeds, and salt.
6. Mix well and pour it into ramekins.
7. Add it to the Air Fryer basket.
8. Place the ramekins inside the Air Fryer and close the lid.
9. Bake it for 8 minutes at 375°F.
10. Once egg muffins are firm, serve and enjoy.

Serving Suggestion: Serve it with toast
Variation tip: Use mozzarella cheese
Nutrition: Calories: 206 | Fats: 14.6 g | Carbs: 7.9 g | Protein: 14.4 g

Easy Asparagus Quiche

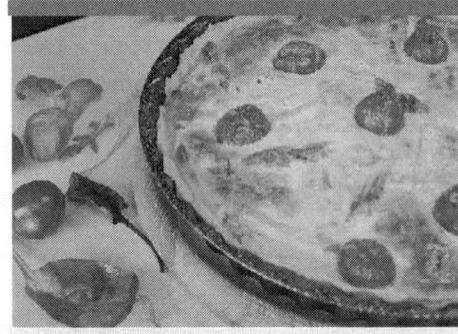

Preparation: 10 min
Cooking: 45 min
Servings: 8

Ingredients:
- 10 eggs
- 2 lbs. asparagus, trimmed and remove ends
- 3 tbsp olive oil
- Pepper, to taste
- 10 Cherry tomatoes, sliced
- Salt, to taste

Directions:
1. Preheat the oven to 425 F.
2. Arrange asparagus on the baking sheet. Drizzle 1 tablespoon olive oil over asparagus.
3. Roast asparagus in preheated oven for 15 minutes.
4. In a mixing bowl, whisk eggs with remaining oil, pepper, tomatoes and salt.
5. Transfer roasted asparagus in a quiche pan. Pour egg mixture over asparagus.
6. Bake at 350 F for 30 minutes or until egg sets.
7. Slice and serve.

Nutrition: Calories 146 g | Fat 10.9 g | Protein 9.4 g |

Balsamic Mushroom and Asparagus

Ingredients:
- 1-pound green beans
- 1-pound mushrooms
- 1-pound asparagus
- 2 teaspoons olive oil
- 1 tablespoon balsamic vinegar
- Salt and pepper

Preparation: 5 min | **Cooking:** 7 min | **Servings:** 2

Directions:
1. Take a medium bowl, and mix all the listed ingredients.
2. Place the vegetables in the Air Fryer basket.
3. Air fry at 400°F for 7 minutes.
4. Shake the vegetables halfway through.
5. Once done, serve.

Serving Suggestion: Serve it with coleslaw
Variation tip: None
Nutrition: Calories:161 | Fats: 5.6 g | Carbs: 23.7 g | Protein: 11.3 g

Crunchy Quinoa Meal

Ingredients:
- 3 cups coconut milk
- 1 cup rinsed quinoa
- 1/8 teaspoons ground cinnamon
- 1 cup raspberry
- ½ cup chopped coconuts

Preparation: 5 min | **Cooking:** 25 min | **Servings:** 2

Directions:
1. In a saucepan, pour milk and bring to a boil over moderate heat.
2. Add the quinoa to the milk and then bring it to a boil once more.
3. Let it simmer for at least 15 minutes on medium heat until the milk is reduced.
4. Stir in the cinnamon, then mix properly.
5. Cover it, then cook for 8 minutes until the milk is completely absorbed.
6. Add the raspberry and cook the meal for 30 seconds.
7. Serve and enjoy.

Nutrition: Calories: 271 | Fats: 3.7 g | Carbs: 54 g | Protein: 6.5 g

Pasta With Indian Lentils

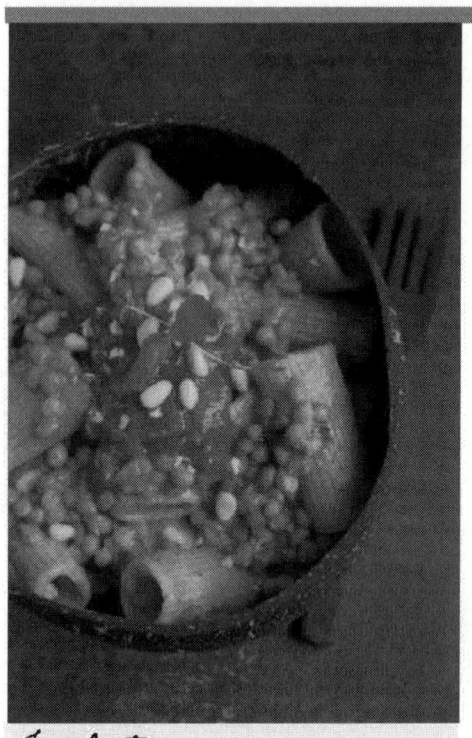

Preparation: 5 min | **Cooking:** 0 min | **Servings:** 6

Directions:
1. Combine all ingredients in the skillet except cilantro, then boil on medium-high heat.
2. Ensure to cover and slightly reduce heat to medium-low and simmer until pasta is tender for about 35 minutes.
3. Afterward, take out the chili peppers and add cilantro.

Nutrition: Calories: 175 | Carbs: 40 g | Protein: 3 g | Fats: 2 g |

Ingredients:
- ¼ - ½ cup fresh cilantro, chopped
- 3 cups water
- 2 small dry red peppers (whole)
- 1 teaspoon turmeric
- 1 teaspoon ground cumin
- 2-3 cloves garlic, minced
- 1 can diced tomatoes (w/juice)
- 1 large onion, chopped
- ½ cup dry lentils, rinsed
- ½ cup orzo or tiny pasta

Cranberry and Roasted Squash Delight

Ingredients:
- ¼ cup chopped walnuts
- ¼ teaspoon thyme
- ½ tablespoon chopped Italian parsley
- 1 cup diced onion
- 1 cup fresh cranberries
- 1 small orange, peeled and segmented
- 2 teaspoons canola oil, divided
- 4 cups cooked wild rice
- 4 cups diced winter squash, peeled and cut into ½-inch cubes
- Pepper to taste

Preparation: 10 min | **Cooking:** 60 min | **Servings:** 8

Directions:
1. Grease the roasting pan with cooking spray and preheat the oven to 400°F.
2. In a roasting pan, place the squash cubes, add a teaspoon of oil, and toss to coat. Place it in the oven and roast until lightly browned, around 40 minutes.
3. Place a nonstick frying pan on a medium-high fire and heat the remaining oil. Once hot, add onions and sauté until lightly browned and tender, around 5 minutes.
4. Add cranberries and continue stir-frying for a minute.
5. Add the remaining ingredients into a pan and cook until heated, around 4 to 5 minutes.
6. Best served warm.

Nutrition: Calories: 166.2 | Protein: 4.8 g | Carbs: 29.1 g | Fats: 3.4 g

Mozzarella Pasta Mix

Ingredients:
- 2 oz whole grain elbow macaroni
- 1 tablespoon fresh basil
- ¼ cup cherry size Mozzarella
- ½ cup cherry tomatoes, halved
- 1 tablespoon olive oil
- 1 teaspoon dried marjoram
- 1 cup water, for cooking

Preparation: 15 min | **Cooking:** 15 min | **Servings:** 2

Directions:
1. Boil elbow macaroni in water for 15 minutes. Drain water and chill macaroni a little.
2. Chop the fresh basil roughly and place it in the salad bowl.
3. Add Mozzarella, cherry tomatoes, dried marjoram, olive oil, and macaroni.
4. Mix up salad well.

Nutrition: Calories 170 | Fats: 9.7 g | Carbs: 15 g | Protein: 6 g

Citrus Quinoa & Chickpea Salad

Ingredients:
- 2 cups cooked quinoa
- 1 can chickpeas, drained and rinsed
- 1 ripe avocado, diced
- 1 red bell pepper, diced
- ½ red onion, diced
- ¼ cup lime juice
- ½ tablespoons garlic powder
- ½ tablespoons paprika
- ¼ - ½ cup chopped cilantro
- 1 tablespoon chopped jalapenos
- Sea salt to taste

Preparation: 10 min | **Cooking:** 0 min | **Servings:** 4

Directions:
1. Add all ingredients to a large bowl and mix well.
2. Enjoy right away or refrigerate for later.

Nutrition: Calories: 300 | Carbs: 43.5 g | Protein: 10.3 g | Fats: 10.9 g

Rosemary Roasted New Potatoes

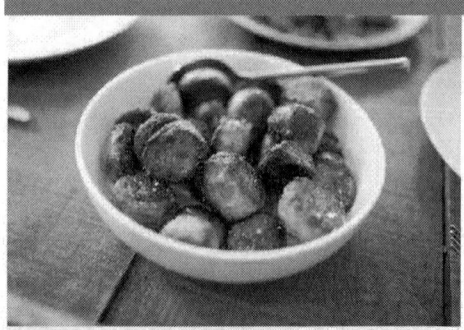

Preparation: 10 min
Cooking: 1 hr 30 min
Servings: 3

Ingredients:

- 2 pounds new potatoes, washed
- 3 tablespoons olive oil
- 2 rosemary sprigs
- 4 garlic cloves, crushed
- Salt and pepper to taste

Directions:

1. Place the new potatoes in a large pot and cover them with water. Cook for 15 minutes, then drain well.
2. Heat the oil in a skillet and add the rosemary and garlic.
3. Stir in the potatoes and continue cooking on a medium flame for 20 minutes or until evenly golden brown.
4. Serve the potatoes warm.

Nutrition : Calories : 168 | Fats: 7.2 g | Protein: 2.7 g | Carbs: 24.6 g

Couscous and Toasted Almonds

Ingredients:

- 1 cup (about 200 g) whole-grain couscous
- 400 ml boiling water
- 1 tablespoon extra-virgin olive oil
- ½ red onion, chopped
- ½ teaspoon ground ginger
- ½ teaspoon ground cinnamon and
- ½ teaspoon ground coriander
- 2 tablespoons blanched almonds, toasted and chopped

Preparation: 5 min
Cooking: 10 min
Servings: 2

Directions:

1. Preheat the oven to 110°C (230F).
2. In a casserole, toss the couscous with olive oil, onion, spices, salt, and pepper.
3. Stir in the boiling water, cover, and bake for 10 minutes.
4. Fluff using a fork. Scatter the nuts over the top and then serve.

Nutrition: Calories: 241.23 | Total fats: 8 g | Carbs: 37 g | Protein: 7 g

Chickpeas and Beets Mix

Ingredients:
- 3 tablespoons capers, drained and chopped
- 1 lemon, juiced
- Zest of 1 lemon, grated
- 1 red onion, chopped
- 3 tablespoons olive oil
- 14 ounces canned chickpeas, drained
- 8 ounces beets, peeled and cubed
- 1 tablespoon parsley, chopped
- Salt and pepper to taste

Preparation: 5 min
Cooking: 25 min
Servings: 2

Directions:
1. Heat a pan with the oil over medium fire. Add the onion, lemon zest, lemon juice, and the capers and sauté for 5 minutes.
2. Add the rest of the ingredients, stir and cook over medium-low heat for 20 minutes.
3. Divide the mix between plates and serve as a side dish.

Nutrition: Calories: 199 | Fats: 4.5 | Carbs: 6.5 | Protein: 3.3

Air Fryer Stuffed Peppers

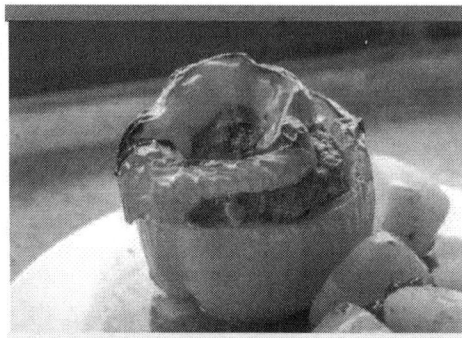

Preparation: 20 min
Cooking: 18 min
Servings: 6

Ingredients:
- 6 bell peppers
- 1 tablespoon olive oil
- 1/3 cup green onion diced
- ¼ cup fresh parsley
- ¼ teaspoon ground sage
- ¼ teaspoon garlic salt
- 1 cup marinara sauce
- ½ cup shredded mozzarella cheese

Directions:
1. Add oil to a skillet.
2. Then add green onion, parsley, sage, and salt.
3. Let it cook for 2 minutes, then add the marinara sauce and mix well.
4. Cut the top off of the bell peppers and clean the cavity.
5. Scoop the skillet mixture into each of the peppers and top with cheese.
6. Place it in the basket of the Air Fryer.
7. Cook for 18 minutes at 355°F.
8. Once done, serve.

Variation tip: Use sesame oil with olive oil
Nutrition: Calories:102 | Fats: 4.2 g | Carbs: 15.1 g | Protein: 2.7 g

Avocado Boat with Salsa

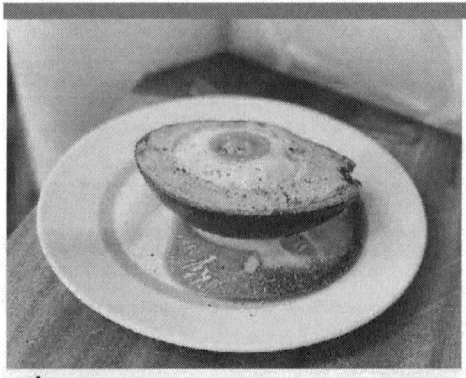

Preparation: 10 min
Cooking: 30 min
Servings: 2

Directions:

1. Preheat the oven to 175°F.
2. Halve the avocado lengthways, remove the stone and brush the flesh with lemon juice.
3. Line a baking sheet with a piece of parchment paper and spread the avocado halves on top. Slide an egg into the core's hollow and sprinkle with a little salt.
4. Bake on the middle rack for 15-20 minutes.
5. In the meantime, prepare the salsa. To do this, peel and finely chop the onion, wash the tomato, and cut it into fine cubes. Mix both with the olive oil and vinegar in a bowl. Season to taste with salt and pepper.
6. Take the avocado out of the oven and serve it with the salsa on two plates.

Nutrition: Calories: 300 | Total Fats: 17 g Total Carbs: 34 g | Protein: 7 g

Ingredients:

- 1 avocado
- 2 medium-sized eggs
- 1 large tomato
- 1 teaspoon lemon juice
- ½ red onion
- 1 teaspoon olive oil
- 1 teaspoon white wine vinegar
- Salt and pepper

Low-Carb Berry Salad With Citrus Dressing

Ingredients:

Salad:
- ¼ cup blueberries
- ½ cup chopped strawberries
- 1 cup mixed greens (kale and chard)
- 2 cups baby spinach
- 2 chopped green onions
- ½ cup chopped avocado
- 1 shredded carrot

Citrus Dressing:
- 1 tablespoon extra-virgin olive oil
- 2 tablespoons apple cider vinegar
- ¼ cup fresh orange juice
- 5 strawberries chopped

Preparation: 10 min
Cooking: 0 min
Servings: 3

Directions:

1. In a blender, blend all dressing ingredients until very smooth; set aside.
2. Combine all salad ingredients in a large bowl; drizzle with dressing, and toss to coat well before serving.

Nutrition: Calories: 300 | Total Fats: 17 g | Total Carbs: 34 g | Protein: 7 g

Spaghetti Squash

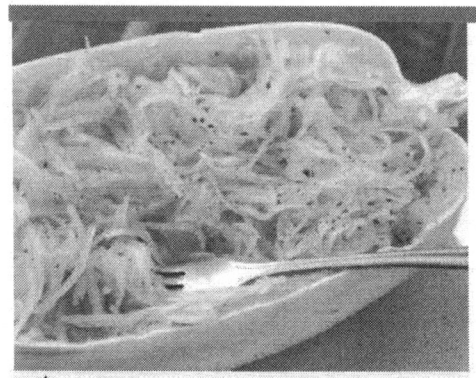

Preparation: 15 min
Cooking: 45 min
Servings: 4

Ingredients:
- 1 spaghetti squash
- 1 pinch black pepper
- 1 tablespoon olive oil
- 1 tablespoon Pecorino Romano, shredded

Directions:
1. Preheat your oven to 425°F.
2. Cut the spaghetti squash in half, remove its seeds, and place it on a baking sheet.
3. Drizzle black pepper and olive oil on top; then bake for 45 minutes.
4. Scrap the squash flesh with a fork and add to the serving plate.
5. Drizzle pecorino Romano on top.
6. Serve.

Variation tip: Add lemon zest and lemon juice for better taste.
Nutrition: Fats: 5 g | Sodium: 432 mg | Carbs: 13.1 g | Protein: 5.7 g

Zucchini and Tomatoes

Preparation: 10 min
Cooking: 8 min
Servings: 3

Ingredients:
- 1 teaspoon garlic cloves, minced
- 1 teaspoon olive oil
- salt, to taste
- 1 teaspoon Stevia
- 1 teaspoon dry basil
- 2 tablespoons parmesan cheese
- 2 cups zucchini, sliced
- ½ cup tomatoes, sliced

Directions:
1. Preheat the Air Fryer to 400°F for 10 minutes.
2. Take a bowl and add olive oil, salt, stevia, minced garlic clove, dry basil, zucchini, and tomatoes.
3. Mix well and add it to the Air Fryer basket.
4. Air fry it for 8 minutes at 350°F.
5. Serve it with parmesan cheese on top.

Serving Suggestion: Serve it with French fries
Variation tip: None
Nutrition: Calories: 62 | Fats: 3.8 g | Carbs: 4.2 g | Protein: 4.2 g

Vegan Meatballs

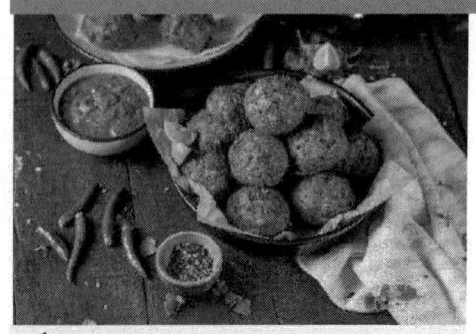

Preparation: 20 min
Cooking: 48 min
Servings: 4

Ingredients:

- 1 cup cooked quinoa
- 1 (15-ounce) can black beans
- 2 tablespoons water
- 3 garlic cloves, minced
- ½ cup shallot, diced
- ¼ teaspoon salt
- 2 ½ teaspoons fresh oregano
- ½ teaspoon red pepper flake
- ½ teaspoon fennel seeds
- ½ cup vegan parmesan cheese, shredded
- 2 tablespoons tomato paste
- 3 tablespoons fresh basil, chopped
- 2 tablespoons Worcestershire sauce

Directions:

1. Preheat your oven to 350°F.
2. Spread the beans on a baking sheet and bake for 15 minutes.
3. Meanwhile, sauté garlic, shallots, and water in a skillet for 3 minutes.
4. Transfer to the food processor along with fennel, red pepper flakes, baked beans, oregano, and salt.
5. Blend these ingredients just until incorporated.
6. Stir in quinoa and the rest of the ingredients, then mix evenly.
7. Make golf-ball-sized meatballs out of this mixture.
8. Spread these meatballs on a greased baking sheet and bake for 20-30 minutes until brown.
9. Flip the meatballs once cooked halfway through.
10. Serve warm.

Serving Suggestion: Serve the meatballs with pita bread and chili sauce.
Nutrition: Calories:338 | Fat 24 g | Carbs: 58.3 g | Protein: 5.4 g

Spinach Alfredo Soup

Ingredients:

- 2 cups cauliflower florets
- ½ teaspoon garlic, minced
- 1 teaspoon olive oil
- ½ cup cottage cheese
- 9 ounces shredded cheese
- 6 wedges light laughing cow cheese
- ½ teaspoon salt
- ¼ teaspoon black pepper
- 1 cup cashew milk
- 26 ounces frozen spinach
- 3 tablespoons parmesan cheese, shredded
- 18 ounces yogurt

Preparation: 15 min
Cooking: 23 min
Servings: 6

Directions:

1. Boil cauliflower in a cooking pan filled with water for 10 minutes.
2. Transfer the cauliflower florets to a blender along with 1 cup of cooking liquid.
3. Puree this mixture and keep it aside.
4. Sauté garlic with olive oil in a suitable pan for 3 minutes.
5. Transfer to the cauliflower and add cheese, black pepper, milk, and salt.
6. Blend these ingredients until smooth.
7. Return the mixture to the saucepan and add one more cup of cooking liquid.
8. Cook the soup to a boil, add spinach, and cook for 10 minutes.
9. Serve warm.

Serving Suggestion: Serve the soup with cauliflower rice.
Variation tip: Add broccoli florets to the soup as well.
Nutrition: Calories: 314 | Fats: 2.2 g | Carbs: 27.7 g | Protein: 8.8 g

Air Fryer Spaghetti Squash

Ingredients:
- 1 (3 pounds) spaghetti squash
- 1 teaspoon olive oil
- ¼ teaspoon sea salt
- 1/8 teaspoon ground black pepper
- 1/8 teaspoon smoked paprika

Preparation: 25 min
Cooking: 25 min
Servings: 6

Directions:
1. Create a dotted line lengthwise around the squash with a knife.
2. Cook the squash in the microwave at high for 5 minutes.
3. Transfer it to a cutting board
4. Cut the squash in half lengthwise,
5. Spoon pulp and seeds out of the one-half and discard.
6. Brush it with olive oil
7. Season it with salt, pepper, and paprika.
8. Preheat the Air Fryer to 360°F
9. Once preheated, put the squash half skin side-down in the basket.
10. Cook for 20 minutes.
11. Serve and enjoy.

Serving Suggestion: Serve it with sour cream
Variation tip: Use oil spray instead of olive oil
Nutrition: Calories:77 | Fats: 2.1 g | Carbs: 15.7 g | Protein: 1.5 g

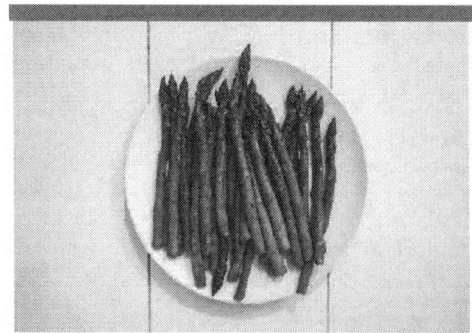

Asparagus With Garlic

Preparation: 15 min
Cooking: 45 min
Servings: 4

Ingredients:
- 1 lb. thick asparagus spears, trimmed and chopped
- ½ cup garlic cloves, peeled and chopped
- 3 tablespoons olive oil
- Salt and black pepper to taste

Directions:
1. Mix asparagus with garlic, olive oil, black pepper, and salt in a bowl.
2. Cover and marinate for 30 minutes.
3. Meanwhile, at 450°F, preheat your oven.
4. Spread the asparagus on a baking sheet.
5. Roast them for 15 minutes in the preheated oven.
6. Serve warm.

Serving Suggestion: Serve the asparagus with toasted bread slices.
Variation tip: Add boiled zucchini pasta to the mixture.
Nutrition: Calories:136 | Fats: 10 g | Carbs: 8 g | Protein: 4 g

Zucchini Lasagna

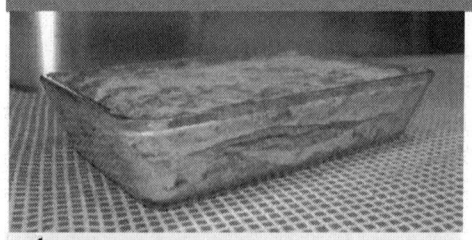

Preparation: 15 min
Cooking: 24 min
Servings: 4

Ingredients:
- 6 ounces crumbled tofu
- 1 garlic clove, minced
- 1 tablespoon dried parsley flakes
- 1 tablespoon dried basil
- 1/8 teaspoons salt
- 1 can diced tomatoes, drained
- ¾ cup 1% cottage cheese, shredded
- 3 ounces fat free mozzarella cheese, shredded
- 1 tablespoon dried parsley flakes
- 2 tablespoons egg, beaten
- 2 small zucchini squash

Directions:
1. At 350°F, preheat your oven.
2. Cut the whole zucchini into thin slices using a potato peeler.
3. Sauté tofu with garlic, parsley, basil, and salt in a cooking pan until golden brown.
4. Stir in tomatoes, egg, and parsley; then cook for 4 minutes.
5. Spread a layer of thin zucchini slices at the bottom of a casserole dish.
6. Top these slices with half of the tofu mixture.
7. Mix cottage cheese with mozzarella cheese in a bowl.
8. Drizzle 1/3 of the cheese mixture over the tofu filling.
9. Repeat the zucchini layer and top it with the remaining tofu mixture.
10. Add 1/3 of the cheese mixture and add another layer of zucchini on top.
11. Drizzle the remaining cheese on top and bake for 20 minutes in the oven.
12. Serve warm.

Serving Suggestion: Serve the lasagna with the spinach salad.
Nutrition: Calories:204 | Fats: 21 g | Carbs: 21.4 g | Protein: 4.6 g

Mexican Cauliflower Rice

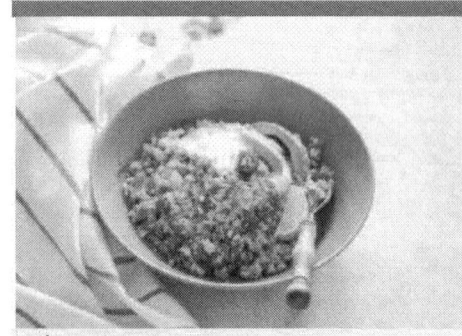

Preparation: 15 min
Cooking: 14 min
Servings: 4

Ingredients:
- 1 head cauliflower, riced
- 1 tablespoon olive oil
- 1 medium white onion, diced
- 2 garlic cloves, minced
- 1 jalapeno, seeded and minced
- 3 tablespoons tomato paste
- 1 teaspoon sea salt
- 1 teaspoon cumin
- ½ teaspoon paprika
- 3 tablespoons fresh cilantro, chopped
- 1 tablespoon lime juice

Directions:
1. Grate the cauliflower in a food processor.
2. Sauté onion with oil in a skillet over medium-high heat for 6 minutes.
3. Stir in jalapeno and garlic, then sauté for 2 minutes.
4. Add paprika, cumin, salt, and tomato paste, then sauté for 1 minute.
5. Stir in cauliflower rice and the rest of the ingredients and cook for 5 minutes.
6. Add cilantro and lime juice to the top.
7. Serve.

Serving Suggestion: Serve the rice with roasted veggies on the side.
Variation tip: Add canned corn to the rice.
Nutrition: Calories: 351 | Fats: 19 g | Carbs: 43 g | Protein: 23 g

Quick Collard Greens

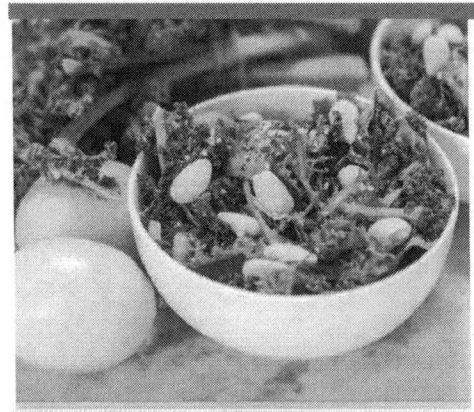

Preparation: 8 min

Cooking: 7 min

Servings: 2

Ingredients:

- 10-ounces collard greens
- 1 ½ tablespoon extra-virgin olive oil
- ¼ teaspoon fine sea salt
- 2 garlic cloves, pressed or minced
- A Pinch red pepper flakes
- A couple lemon wedges for serving

Directions:

For preparing the collard:

1. Slice the thick center rib out of each collard green.
2. Stack the rib-less green and roll it up into a cigar-like shape.
3. Cut "cigar" thinly to prepare long strands.
4. Place the skillet on the stove over a medium-high flame and add olive oil.
5. When shimmering, add the salt and all collard green.
6. Stir well until all greens are coated with oil and cook for half-minute.
7. Stir well and cook for half-minute more until dark green, greens are wilted, and brown on the edges. It will take 3 to 6 minutes.
8. When done, add red pepper flakes and garlic. Cook for half-minute until fragrant.
9. Remove from the pan and the flame.
10. Split cooked collard on the serving plate.
11. Serve with a lemon wedge and almonds

Variation tip: If you don't want to add spice, skip red pepper flakes.
Serving Suggestion: Serve with a lemon wedge.
Nutrition: Calories: 110 | Fats: 6.4 g | Carbs: 8.8 g | Protein: 4.5 g

Grains, Beans & Legumes

Chapter 5

Black Eyed Peas Stew

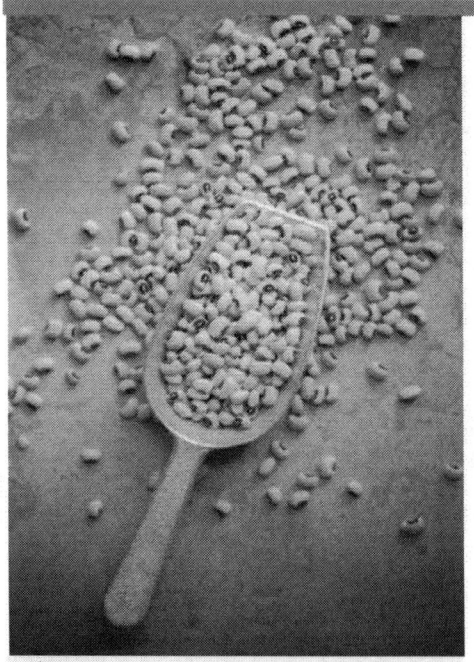

Preparation: 10 min | **Cooking:** 20 min | **Servings:** 4

Directions:

1. Heat a pot on a medium-high fire. Add ¼ cup of oil and heat for 3 minutes.
2. Stir in bay leaves and tomato paste. Sauté for 2 minutes.
3. Stir in carrots and a cup of water. Cover and simmer for 5 minutes.
4. Stir in dill, parsley, beans, and orange. Cover and cook for 3 minutes or until heated through.
5. Season with pepper and salt to taste.
6. Stir in the remaining oil and green onions and cook for 2 minutes.
7. Serve and enjoy.

Nutrition: Calories: 376 | Protein: 8.8 g | Carbs: 25.6 g | Fats: 27.8 g

Ingredients:

- ½ cup extra virgin olive oil, divided
- 1 cup fresh dill, stems removed, chopped
- 1 cup fresh parsley, stems removed, chopped
- 1 cup water
- 2 bay leaves
- 2 carrots, peeled and sliced
- 2 cups black-eyed beans, drained and rinsed
- 2 slices orange with peel and flesh
- 2 tablespoons tomato paste
- 4 green onions, thinly sliced
- Salt and pepper to taste

Chickpea Alfredo Sauce

Preparation: 10 min | **Cooking:** 0 min | **Servings:** 4

Ingredients:

- ¼ teaspoon ground nutmeg
- ¼ teaspoon sea salt or to taste
- 1 clove garlic minced
- 2 cups chickpeas, rinsed and drained
- 1 tablespoon white miso paste
- 1 - ½ cups water
- 2 tablespoons lemon juice
- 3 tablespoons nutritional yeast

Directions:

1. Add all ingredients to a blender.
2. Puree until smooth and creamy.

Nutrition: Calories: 123 | Protein: 6.2 g | Carbs: 20.2 g | Fats: 2.4 g

Chickpea Eggplant Salad

Ingredients:
- 1 cup chopped dill
- 1 cup chopped parsley
- 1 cup cooked or canned chickpeas, drained
- 1 large eggplant, thinly sliced (no more than ¼ inch in thickness)
- 1 small red onion, sliced in ½ moons
- ½ English cucumber, diced
- 3 Roma tomatoes, diced
- 3 tablespoons Za'atar spice, divided
- Oil for frying, preferably extra virgin olive oil
- Salt

Garlic Vinaigrette Ingredients:
- 1 large lime, juiced
- 1/3 cup extra virgin olive oil
- 1 - 2 garlic cloves, minced
- Salt and Pepper to taste

Preparation: 10 min
Cooking: 10 min
Servings: 4

Directions:
1. On a baking sheet, spread out sliced eggplant and season with salt generously. Let it sit for 30 minutes. Then pat dry with a paper towel.
2. Place a small pot on medium-high fire, fill it halfway with oil, and heat oil for 5 minutes. Fry eggplant in batches until golden brown, around 3 minutes per side. Place cooked eggplants on a paper towel-lined plate.
3. Once the eggplants have cooled, assemble them on a serving dish. Sprinkle with 1 tablespoon of Za'atar.
4. Mix dill, parsley, red onions, chickpeas, cucumbers, and tomatoes in a large salad bowl. Sprinkle the remaining Za'atar and gently toss to mix.
5. Whisk well the vinaigrette ingredients in a small bowl. Drizzle 2 tablespoons of the dressing over the steamed eggplant. Add the remaining dressing over the chickpea salad and mix.
6. Add the chickpea salad to the serving dish with the steamed eggplant.
7. Serve and enjoy.

Nutrition: Calories: 642 | Protein: 16.6 g | Carbs: 25.9 g | Fats: 44.0 g

Extraordinary Green Hummus

Ingredients:
- ¼ cup fresh lemon juice (about 1 large lemon's worth)
- ¼ cup roughly chopped, loosely packed fresh tarragon or basil
- ¼ cup tahini
- ½ cup roughly chopped, loosely packed fresh parsley
- ½ teaspoon salt, more to taste
- 1 large garlic clove, roughly chopped
- 1 to 2 tablespoons water, optional
- 2 tablespoons olive oil, plus more for serving
- 2 to 3 tablespoons roughly chopped fresh chives or green onion
- Garnish with extra olive oil and a sprinkling of chopped fresh herbs
- 1 (15-ounce) can of chickpeas, also called garbanzo beans, drained and rinsed

Preparation: 10 min
Cooking: 0 min
Servings: 8

Directions:
1. Place all ingredients in a blender and puree until smooth and creamy.
2. Transfer to a bowl and adjust seasoning if needed.
3. Serve with pita chips.

Nutrition: Calories: 8 | Protein: 3.8 g | Carbs: 10.0 g | Fats: 8.3 g

Bell Peppers 'N Tomato-Chickpea Rice

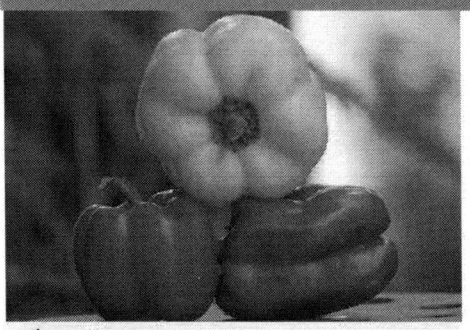

Preparation: 10 min

Cooking: 35 min

Servings: 4

Ingredients:

- 2 tablespoons olive oil
- ½ chopped red bell pepper
- ½ chopped green bell pepper
- ½ chopped yellow pepper
- ½ chopped red pepper
- 1 medium onion, chopped
- 1 clove garlic, minced
- 2 cups cooked jasmine rice
- 1 teaspoon tomato paste
- 1 cup chickpeas
- Salt to taste
- ½ teaspoon paprika
- 1 small tomato, chopped
- Parsley for garnish

Directions:

1. In a large mixing bowl, whisk well olive oil, garlic, tomato paste, and paprika. Season with salt generously.
2. Mix in rice and toss well to coat in the dressing.
3. Add the remaining ingredients and toss well to mix.
4. Let the salad rest to allow flavors to mix for 15 minutes.
5. Toss one more time and adjust salt to taste if needed.
6. Garnish with parsley and serve.

Nutrition: Calories: 490 | Carbs: 93.0 g | Protein: 10.0 g | Fats: 8.0 g

Spaghetti in Lemon Avocado White Sauce

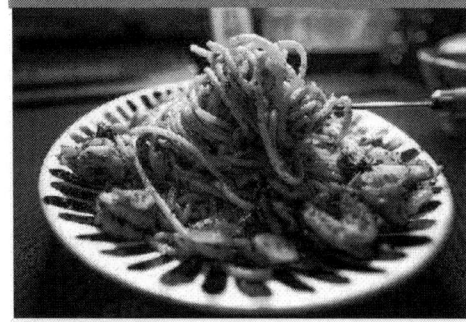

Preparation: 10 min

Cooking: 30 min

Servings: 3

Ingredients:

- Freshly ground black pepper
- 1 lemon zest and juice
- 1 avocado, pitted and peeled
- 1-pound spaghetti
- Salt
- 1 tablespoon olive oil
- 8 oz small shrimp, shelled and deveined
- ¼ cup dry white wine
- 1 large onion, finely sliced

Directions:

1. Let a big pot of water boil. Once boiling, add the spaghetti or pasta and cook following the manufacturer's instructions until al dente. Drain and set aside.
2. In a large frying pan, over medium fire, sauté wine and onions for ten minutes or until onions are translucent and soft.
3. Add the shrimps into the frying pan and increase the fire to high while constantly sautéing until the shrimps are cooked, around 5 minutes. Turn the fire off. Season with salt and add the oil right away. Then quickly toss in the cooked pasta and mix well.
4. In a blender puree the lemon juice and avocado until smooth. Pour into the frying pan of pasta, and combine well. Garnish with pepper and lemon zest, then serve.

Nutrition: Calories: 206 | Carbs: 26.3 g | Protein: 10.2 g | Fats: 8.0 g

Kidney Beans and Beet Salad

Ingredients:

- 1 14.5-ounce can kidney beans, drained and rinsed
- 1 tablespoon pomegranate syrup or juice
- 2 tablespoons olive oil
- 4 beets, scrubbed and stems removed
- 4 green onions, chopped
- 1 lemon, juiced
- Salt and pepper to taste

Preparation: 10 min

Cooking: 15 min

Servings: 3

Directions:

1. Bring a pot of water to boil and add the beets. Simmer for 10 minutes or until tender. Drain the beets and place them in an ice bath for 5 minutes.
2. Peel the bets and slice them in halves.
3. Toss to mix the pomegranate syrup, olive oil, lemon juice, green onions, and kidney beans in a salad bowl.
4. Stir in the beets. Season with pepper and salt to taste.
5. Serve and enjoy.

Nutrition: Calories: 175 | Protein: 6.0 g | Carbs: 22.0 g | Fats: 7.0 g

Kidney Beans and Parsley-lemon Salad

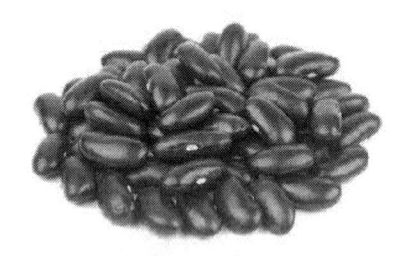

Preparation: 10 min

Cooking: 0 min

Servings: 6

Directions:

1. Whisk well in a small bowl the pepper flakes, salt, garlic, and lemon juice until emulsified.
2. In a serving bowl, combine the red kidney beans, chickpeas, onion, celery, cucumber, parsley, and dill (or mint).
3. Drizzle the salad with the dressing and toss well to coat.
4. Serve and enjoy.

Nutrition: Calories: 228 | Protein: 8.5 g | Carbs: 26.2 g | Fats: 11.0 g

Ingredients:

- ¼ cup lemon juice (about 1 ½ lemon)
- ¼ cup olive oil
- ¾ cup chopped fresh parsley
- ¾ teaspoon salt
- 1 can (15 ounces) chickpeas, rinsed and drained, or 1 ½ cups cooked chickpeas
- 1 medium cucumber, peeled, seeded, and diced
- 1 small red onion, diced
- 2 cans (15 ounces each) red kidney beans, rinsed and drained, or 3 cups cooked kidney beans
- 2 stalks celery, sliced in half or thirds lengthwise and chopped
- 2 tablespoons chopped fresh dill or mint
- 3 cloves garlic, pressed or minced
- Small pinch red pepper flakes

Italian White Bean Soup

Ingredients:

- 1 (14-ounce) can chicken broth
- 1 bunch fresh spinach, rinsed and thinly sliced
- 1 garlic clove, minced
- 1 stalk celery, chopped
- 1 tablespoon lemon juice
- 1 tablespoon vegetable oil
- 1 onion, chopped
- ¼ teaspoon ground black pepper
- 1/8 teaspoon dried thyme
- 2 (16-ounce) cans white kidney beans, rinsed and drained
- 2 cups water

Preparation: 10 min
Cooking: 50 min
Servings: 4

Directions:

1. Place a pot on medium-high fire and heat for 1 minute. Add oil and heat for another minute.
2. Stir in celery and onion. Sauté for 7 minutes.
3. Stir in garlic and cook for another minute.
4. Add water, thyme, pepper, chicken broth, and beans. Cover and simmer for 15 minutes.
5. Remove 2 cups of the bean and celery mixture with a slotted spoon and set aside.
6. With an immersion blender, puree the remaining soup in the pot until smooth and creamy.
7. Return the 2 cups of bean mixture. Stir in spinach and lemon juice. Cook for 2 minutes until heated through and spinach is wilted.
8. Serve and enjoy.

Nutrition: Calories: 245 | Protein: 12.0 g | Carbs: 38.1 g | Fats: 4.9 g

Sicilian-Style Zoodle Spaghetti

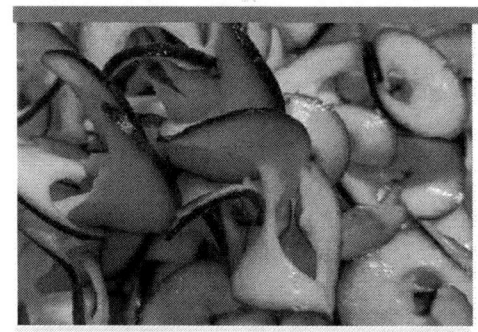

Ingredients:

- 4 cups zoodles (spiraled zucchini)
- 2 ounces cubed vegetarian bacon
- 4 ounces canned sardines, chopped
- ½ cup canned chopped tomatoes
- 1 tablespoon capers
- 1 tablespoon parsley
- 1 teaspoon minced garlic

Preparation: 5 min
Cooking: 10 min
Servings: 2

Directions:

1. Pour some of the sardine oil into a pan.
2. Add garlic and cook for 1 minute.
3. Add the bacon and cook for 2 more minutes.
4. Stir in the tomatoes and let simmer for 5 minutes.
5. Add zoodles and sardines and cook for 3 minutes.

Nutrition: Calories 172 | Fat: 4 g | Carbs: 3 g | Protein: 34 g

Tasty Lime Cilantro Cauliflower Rice

Ingredients:
- 1 head cauliflower, rinsed
- 1 tablespoon extra-virgin olive oil
- 2 garlic cloves, minced
- 2 scallions, chopped
- ½ teaspoon sea salt
- A pinch pepper
- 4 tablespoons fresh lime juice
- ¼ cup chopped fresh cilantro

Preparation: 10 min
Cooking: 10 min
Servings: 3

Directions:
1. Chop the cauliflower and transfer it to a food processor; pulse into a rice texture.
2. Heat a large skillet over medium fire and add olive oil; sauté garlic and scallions for about 4 minutes or until fragrant and tender.
3. Increase heat to medium-high and stir in cauliflower rice; cook covered for about 6 minutes or until cauliflower is crispy on the outside and soft inside.
4. Season with salt and pepper and transfer to a bowl. Toss with freshly squeezed lime juice and cilantro and serve right away.

Nutrition: Calories: 300 | Total Fats: 17 g | Total Carbs: 34 g | Protein: 7 g

Fennel Wild Rice Risotto

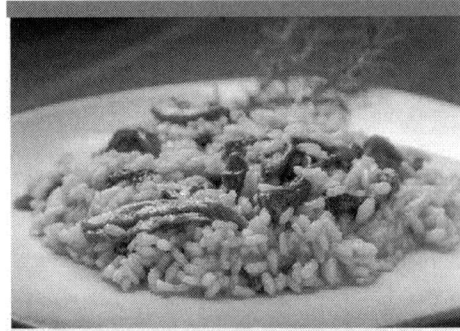

Preparation: 5 min
Cooking: 35 min
Servings: 6

Ingredients:
- 2 tablespoons extra virgin olive oil
- 1 shallot, chopped
- 2 garlic cloves, minced
- 1 fennel bulb, chopped
- 1 cup wild rice
- ¼ cup dry white wine
- 2 cups chicken stock
- 1 teaspoon grated orange zest
- Salt and pepper to taste

Directions:
1. Heat the oil in a heavy saucepan.
2. Add the garlic, shallot, and fennel and cook for a few minutes until softened.
3. Stir in the rice and cook for 2 additional minutes, then add the wine, stock, orange zest, salt, and pepper to taste.
4. Cook on low heat for 20 minutes.
5. Serve the risotto warm and fresh.

Nutrition: Calories: 162 | Fats: 2 g | Protein: 8 g | Carbs: 20 g

Wild Rice Prawn Salad

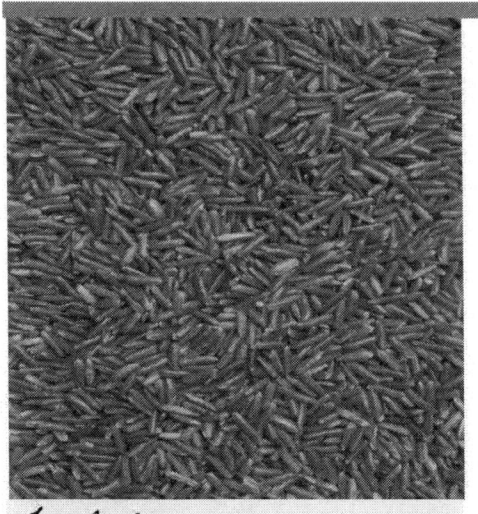

Preparation: 5 min
Cooking: 35 min
Servings: 6

Directions:

1. Combine the rice and chicken stock in a saucepan and cook until the liquid has been absorbed entirely.
2. Transfer the rice to a salad bowl.
3. Season the prawns with salt and pepper and drizzle them with lemon juice and oil.
4. Heat a grill pan over medium flame.
5. Place the prawns on the hot pan and cook on each side for 2-3 minutes.
6. For the salad, combine the rice with arugula and prawns and mix well.
7. Serve the salad fresh.

Nutrition: Calories: 207 | Fats: 4 g | Protein : 20.6 g | Carbs: 17 g

Ingredients:

- ¾ cup wild rice
- 1 ¾ cups chicken stock
- 1-pound prawns
- Salt and pepper to taste
- 2 tablespoons lemon juice
- 2 tablespoons extra virgin olive oil
- 2 cups arugula

White Bean Soup

Ingredients:

- 1 cup celery, chopped
- 1 cup carrots, chopped
- 1 yellow onion, chopped
- 6 cups veggie stock
- 4 garlic cloves, minced
- 2 cup navy beans, dried
- ½ teaspoon basil, dried
- ½ teaspoon sage, dried
- 1 teaspoon thyme, dried
- A pinch of salt and black pepper

Preparation: 10 min
Cooking: 8 hrs 30 min
Servings: 6

Directions:

1. In your slow cooker, combine the beans, stock, and the rest of the ingredients; put the lid on and cook on Low for 8 hours.
2. Divide the soup into bowls and serve right away.

Nutrition: Calories: 264 | Fats: 17.5 g| Carbs: 23.7 g| Protein: 11.5 g

Black Bean Hummus

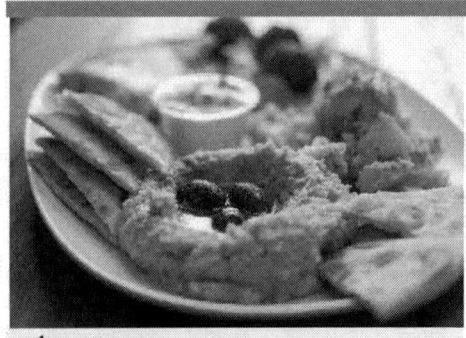

Preparation: 10 min **Cooking:** 0 min **Servings:** 8

Ingredients:
- 10 Greek olives
- ¼ teaspoon paprika
- ¼ teaspoon cayenne pepper
- ½ teaspoon salt
- ¾ teaspoon ground cumin
- 1 ½ tablespoon tahini
- 2 tablespoons lemon juice
- 1 15-oz can black beans, drain and reserve liquid
- 1 clove garlic

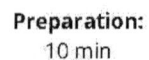

Directions:
1. In a food processor, mince garlic.
2. Add cayenne pepper, salt, cumin, tahini, lemon juice, 2 tablespoons of reserved black beans liquid, and black beans.
3. Process until smooth and creamy. Scrape the side of the processor as needed and continue pureeing.
4. To serve, garnish with Greek olives and paprika.
5. Best eaten as a dip for pita bread or chips.

Nutrition: Calories: 205 | Protein: 12.1 g | Carbs: 34.4 g | Fats: 2.9 g

Brussels Sprouts 'N White Bean Medley

Preparation: 10 min **Cooking:** 15 min **Servings:** 4

Ingredients:
- 1 teaspoon salt
- 2 tablespoon olive oil
- 3 cans white beans, drained and rinsed
- 3 medium onions, peeled and sliced
- 3 tablespoons lemon juice
- 4 ½ cups Brussels sprouts, cleaned and sliced in half
- 6 garlic cloves, smashed, peeled, and minced
- Pepper to taste

Directions:
1. Place a saucepan on medium-high fire and heat for 2 minutes.
2. Add oil and heat for a minute.
3. Sauté garlic and onions for 3 minutes.
4. Stir in Brussels sprouts and sauté for 5 minutes.
5. Stir in white beans and sauté for 5 minutes.
6. Season with pepper and salt.

Nutrition: Calories: 371 | Protein: 21.4 g | Carbs: 57.8 g | Fats: 8.1 g

Chicken and White Beans

Ingredients:

- 2 tablespoons fresh cilantro, chopped
- 3 cups water
- 1/8 teaspoon cayenne pepper
- 2 teaspoons pure chili powder
- 2 teaspoons ground cumin
- 1 (4-ounce) can chopped green chiles
- 1 cup corn kernels
- 2 (15-ounce) cans white beans, drained and rinsed
- 2 garlic cloves
- 1 medium onion, diced
- 2 tablespoons extra-virgin olive oil
- 1 lb. chicken breasts, boneless and skinless

Preparation: 10 min
Cooking: 70 min
Servings: 8

Directions:

1. Slice chicken breasts into ½-inch cubes, and with pepper and salt, season them.
2. On high fire, place a large nonstick frying pan and heat oil.
3. Sauté chicken pieces for three to four minutes or until lightly browned.
4. Reduce fire to medium and add garlic and onion.
5. Cook for 5 to 6 minutes or until the onion is translucent.
6. Add water, spices, chilies, corn, and beans. Bring to a boil.
7. Once boiling, lower the fire and simmer for an hour, uncovered.
8. To serve, garnish with a sprinkling of cilantro and a tablespoon of cheese.

Nutrition: Calories: 433 | Protein: 30.6 g | Carbs: 29.5 g | Fats: 21.8 g

Cilantro-Dijon Vinaigrette on Kidney Beans Salad

Ingredients:

- 1 (15-ounce) can kidney beans, drained and rinsed
- ½ English cucumbers, chopped
- 1 medium-sized heirloom tomato, chopped
- 1 bunch fresh cilantro, stems removed, chopped (about 1 ¼ cup)
- 1 red onion, chopped (about 1 cup)

Cilantro-Dijon Vinaigrette Ingredients:

- 1 large lemon, juiced
- 3 tablespoon olive oil
- 1 teaspoon Dijon mustard
- ½ teaspoon fresh garlic paste or finely chopped garlic
- 1 teaspoon sumac
- Salt and pepper to taste

Directions:

1. In a small bowl, mix well all vinaigrette ingredients.
2. In a salad bowl, combine cilantro, chopped veggies, and kidney beans.
3. Add vinaigrette to the salad and toss well to mix.
4. For 30 minutes, allow flavors to mix and set in the fridge.
5. Mix and adjust seasoning if needed before serving.

Nutrition: Calories: 154 | Protein: 5.5 g | Carbs: 18.3 g | Fats: 7.4 g

Chickpea Salad Moroccan Style

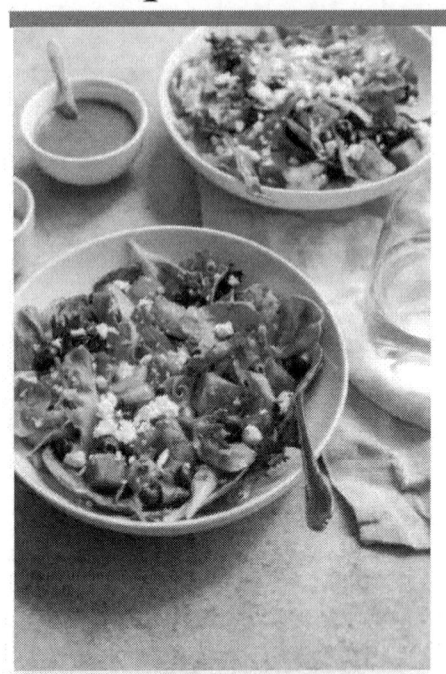

Preparation:	Cooking:	Servings:
10 min	10 min	6

Directions:

1. Make the dressing by whisking cayenne, black pepper, salt, cumin, lemon juice, and oil in a small bowl and set aside.
2. Mix feta, mint, cilantro, red pepper, tomatoes, onions, carrots, and chickpeas in a large salad bowl.
3. Pour dressing over salad and toss to coat well.
4. Serve and enjoy.

Nutrition: Calories: 300 | Protein: 13.2 g | Carbs: 35.4 g | Fats: 12.8 g

Ingredients:

- 1/3 cup crumbled low-fat feta cheese
- ¼ cup fresh mint, chopped
- ¼ cup fresh cilantro, chopped
- 1 red bell pepper, diced
- 2 plum tomatoes, diced
- 3 green onions, sliced thinly
- 1 large carrot, peeled and julienned
- 3 cups BPA-free canned chickpeas or garbanzo beans
- A pinch cayenne pepper
- ¼ teaspoon salt
- ¼ teaspoon pepper
- 2 teaspoons ground cumin
- 3 tablespoons fresh lemon juice
- 3 tablespoon olive oil

White Bean Smoothie to Burn Fats

Ingredients:

- 1 cup unsweetened rice milk (chilled)
- ¼ cup peach slices
- ¼ cup white beans, cooked
- A pinch cinnamon powder
- A pinch nutmeg

Preparation:	Cooking:	Servings:
10 min	0 min	2

Directions:

1. Pour milk into the blender and add the other ingredients to blend till smooth enough to serve and drink.

Nutrition: Calories: 335 | Fats: 3 g | Fiber: 5 g | Carbs: 28 g | Protein: 9 g

BEEF PORK & LAMB

Chapter 6

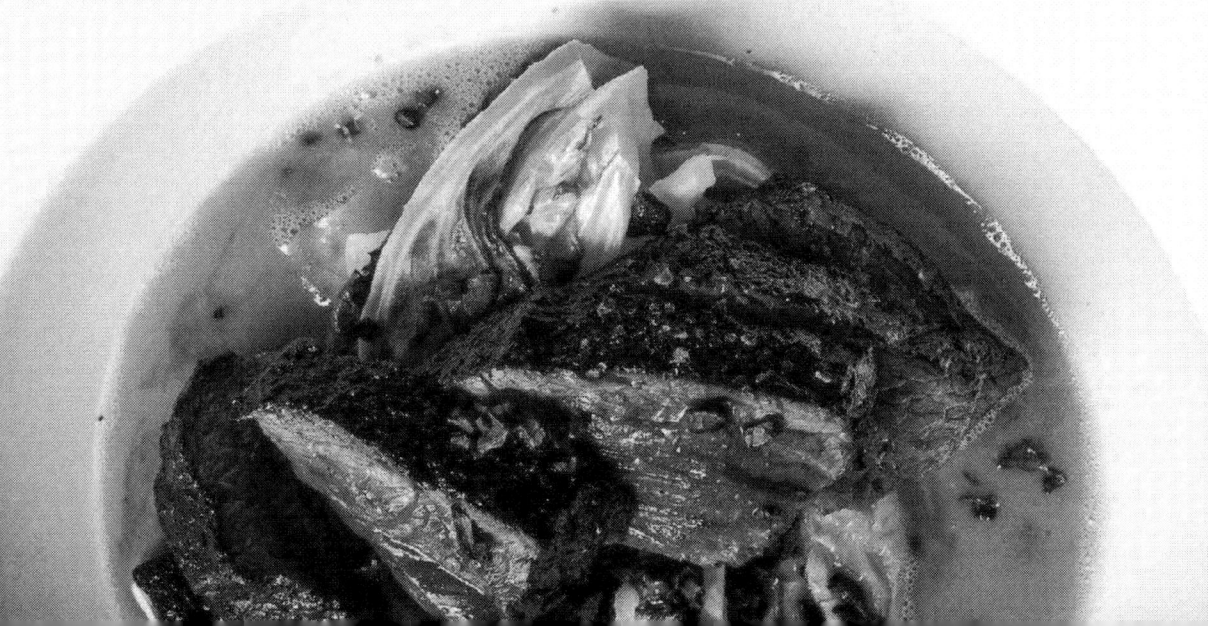

Although red meat is not recommended for those suffering from NAFLD, it is possible to cook it simply and lightly to ensure not to overload the liver, for this reason, we added this chapter with some recipes suitable for you. Enjoy!

Hot Pork Meatballs

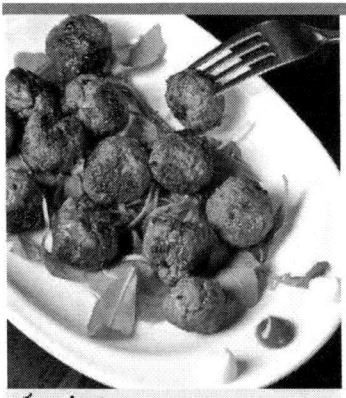

Preparation: 10 min
Cooking: 10 min
Servings: 3

Directions:

1. Mix the ground meat, garlic powder, cayenne pepper, ground black pepper, white pepper, and water.
2. With the help of your fingertips, make the small meatballs.
3. Heat olive oil in the skillet.
4. Arrange the meatballs in the oil and cook them for 10 minutes. Flip the meatballs on another side from time to time.

Nutrition: Calories: 162 | Fats: 10.3 g| Carbs: 1 g | Protein: 15.7 g

Ingredients:

- 4 ounces pork loin, grinded
- ½ teaspoon garlic powder
- ¼ teaspoon chili powder
- ¼ teaspoon cayenne pepper
- ¼ teaspoon ground black pepper
- ¼ teaspoon white pepper
- 1 tablespoon water
- 1 teaspoon olive oil

Tasty Lamb Ribs

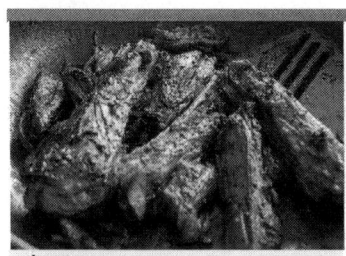

Preparation: 10 min
Cooking: 30 min
Servings: 4

Directions:

1. In a roasting pan, combine the lamb, garlic, shallots, and the rest of the ingredients. Toss, introduce in the oven at 300°F, and cook for 2 hours.
2. Divide the lamb between plates and serve with a side salad.

Nutrition: Calories: 293 | Fats: 9.1 g | Carbs: 16.7 g | Protein: 24.2 g

Ingredients:

- 2 garlic cloves, minced
- ¼ cup shallot, chopped
- 2 tablespoons fish sauce
- ½ cup veggie stock
- 2 tablespoons olive oil
- 1 and ½ tablespoons lemon juice
- 1 tablespoon coriander seeds, ground
- 1 tablespoon ginger, grated
- Salt and black pepper to taste
- 2 pounds lamb ribs

Beef Spread

Ingredients:
- 8 ounces beef liver
- ½ onion, peeled
- ½ carrot, peeled
- ½ teaspoon peppercorns
- 1 bay leaf
- ½ teaspoon salt
- 1/3 cup water
- 1 teaspoon ground black pepper

Preparation: 10 min
Cooking: 25 min
Servings: 3

Directions:
1. Chop the beef liver and put it in the saucepan.
2. Add onion, carrot, peppercorns, bay leaf, salt, and ground black pepper.
3. Add water and close the lid.
4. Boil the beef liver for 25 minutes or until all ingredients are tender.
5. Transfer the cooked mixture to the blender and blend it until smooth.
6. Then place the cooked pate in the serving bowl and flatten the surface of it.
7. Refrigerate the pate for 20-30 minutes before serving.

Nutrition: Calories: 109 | Fats: 2.7 g | Carbs: 5.3 g | Protein: 15.3 g

Pork Chops and Relish

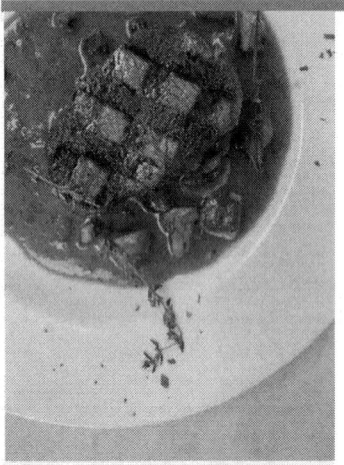

Preparation: 10 min
Cooking: 14 min
Servings: 3

Directions:
1. In a bowl, mix the chops with the pepper sauce, and reserve the liquid from the artichokes. Cover and keep in the fridge for 15 minutes.
2. Heat a grill over medium-high flame. Add the pork chops and cook for 7 minutes on each side.
3. In a bowl, combine the artichokes, peppers, and the remaining ingredients. Toss, divide on top of the chops, and serve.

Nutrition: Calories:215 | Fats: 6 g | Carbs: 6 g | Protein: 35 g

Ingredients:
- 6 pork chops, boneless
- 7 ounces marinated artichoke hearts, chopped and their liquid reserved
- A pinch salt and black pepper
- 1 teaspoon hot pepper sauce
- 1 and ½ cups tomatoes, cubed
- 1 jalapeno pepper, chopped
- ½ cup roasted bell peppers, chopped
- ½ cup black olives, pitted and sliced

Lamb and Tomato Sauce

Ingredients:
- 9 ounces lamb shanks
- 1 onion, diced
- 1 carrot, diced
- 1 tablespoon olive oil
- 1 teaspoon salt
- 1 teaspoon ground black pepper
- 1 ½ cup chicken stock
- 1 tablespoon tomato paste

Preparation: 10 min
Cooking: 55 min
Servings: 3

Directions:
1. Sprinkle the lamb shanks with salt and ground black pepper.
2. Heat olive oil in the saucepan.
3. Add lamb shanks and roast them for 5 minutes from each side.
4. Transfer the meat to the plate.
5. After this, add onion and carrot to the saucepan.
6. Roast the vegetables for 3 minutes.
7. Add tomato paste and mix up well.
8. Then add chicken stock and bring the liquid to a boil.
9. Add lamb shanks, stir well, and close the lid.
10. Cook the meat for 40 minutes over medium-low fire.

Nutrition: Calories: 232 | Fats: 11.3 g| Carbs: 7.3 g| Protein: 25.1 g

Lemony Lamb and Potatoes

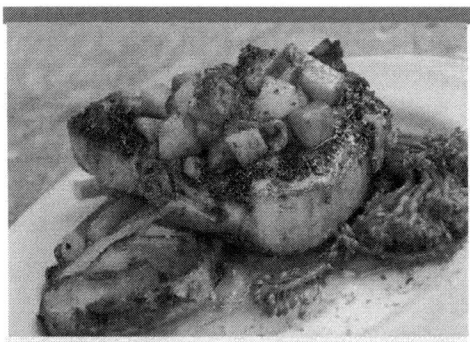

Ingredients:
- 2-pound lamb meat, cubed
- 2 tablespoons olive oil
- 2 springs rosemary, chopped
- 2 tablespoons parsley, chopped
- 1 tablespoon lemon rind, grated
- 3 garlic cloves, minced
- 2 tablespoons lemon juice
- 2 pounds baby potatoes, scrubbed and halved
- 1 cup veggie stock

Preparation: 10 min
Cooking: 2 hrs 10 min
Servings: 3

Directions:
1. In a roasting pan, combine the meat, oil, and the rest of the ingredients. Put them in the oven and bake at 400°F for 2 hours and 10 minutes.
2. Divide the mix between plates and serve.

Nutrition: Calories: 302 | Fats: 15.2 g| Carbs: 23.3g | Protein: 35.2 g

Cumin Lamb Mix

Ingredients:
- 2 lamb chops (3.5-ounce each)
- 1 tablespoon olive oil
- 1 teaspoon ground cumin
- ½ teaspoon salt

Preparation: 10 min
Cooking: 30 min
Servings: 3

Directions:
1. Rub the lamb chops with ground cumin and salt.
2. Then sprinkle them with olive oil.
3. Let the meat marinate for 10 minutes.
4. After this, preheat the skillet well.
5. Place the lamb chops in the skillet and roast them for 10 minutes. Flip the meat on another side from time to time to avoid burning.

Nutrition: Calories: 384 | Fats: 33.2 g| Carbs: 0.5 g | Protein: 19.2 g

Pork and Figs Mix

Ingredients:
- 3 tablespoons avocado oil
- 1 and ½ pounds pork stew meat, roughly cubed
- Salt and black pepper to taste
- 1 cup red onions, chopped
- 1 cup figs, dried and chopped
- 1 tablespoon ginger, grated
- 1 tablespoon garlic, minced
- 1 cup canned tomatoes, crushed
- 2 tablespoons parsley, chopped

Preparation: 10 min
Cooking: 40 min
Servings: 3

Directions:
1. Heat a pot with the oil over a medium-high fire. Add the meat and brown for 5 minutes.
2. Add the onions and sauté for 5 minutes more.
3. Add the rest of the ingredients, bring to a simmer and cook over medium heat for 30 minutes more.
4. Divide the mix between plates and serve.

Nutrition: Calories: 309 | Fats: 16g | Carbs: 21.1 g| Protein: 34.2 g

Greek Style Lamb Chops

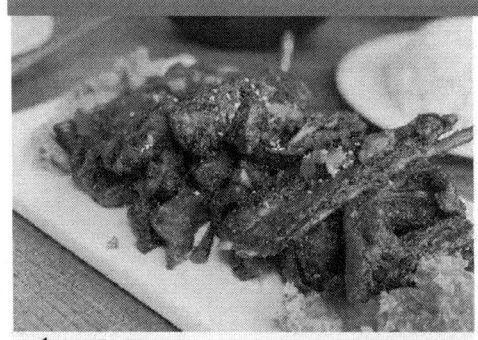

Preparation: 10 min
Cooking: 4 min
Servings: 3

Ingredients:
- ¼ teaspoon black pepper
- ½ teaspoon salt
- 1 tablespoon bottled minced garlic
- 1 tablespoon dried oregano
- 2 tablespoons lemon juice
- 8 pieces lamb loin chops, around 4 ounces
- Cooking spray

Directions:
1. Preheat broiler.
2. In a big bowl or dish, combine the black pepper, salt, minced garlic, lemon juice, and oregano. Then rub it equally on all sides of the lamb chops.
3. Then coat a broiler pan with the cooking spray before placing the lamb chops on the pan and broiling until the desired doneness is reached or for four minutes.

Nutrition: Calories: 131.9 | Carbs: 2.6 g | Protein: 17.1 g | Fats: 5.9 g

Pork and Peas

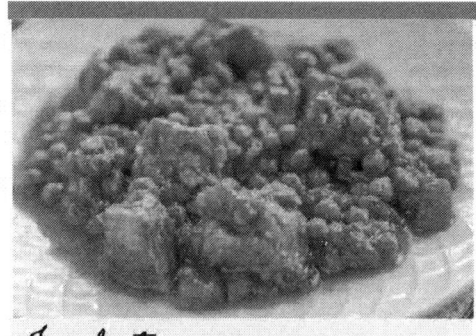

Preparation: 10 min
Cooking: 30 min
Servings: 3

Ingredients:
- 4 ounces snow peas
- 2 tablespoons avocado oil
- 1 pound pork loin, boneless and cubed
- ¾ cup beef stock
- ½ cup red onion, chopped
- Salt and white pepper to taste

Directions:
1. Heat a pan with the oil over a medium-high fire. Add the pork and brown for 5 minutes.
2. Add the peas and the rest of the ingredients, toss, bring to a simmer and cook over medium heat for 15 minutes.
3. Divide the mix between plates and serve right away.

Nutrition: Calories: 332 | Fats: 16.5 g| Fiber: 10.3g | Carbs: 20.7 g| Protein: 26.5 g

Pork and Sage Couscous

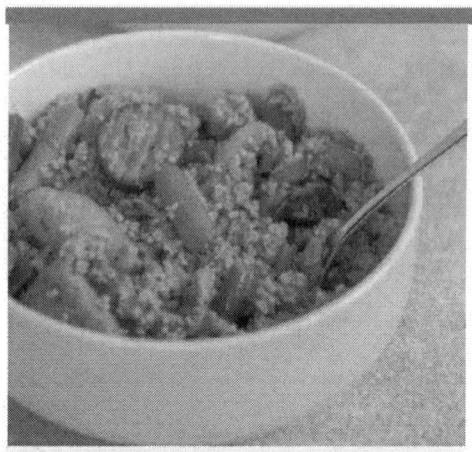

Preparation: 10 min
Cooking: 8 min
Servings: 3

Directions:

1. In a slow cooker, combine the pork, stock, oil, and the other ingredients except for the couscous; put the lid on and cook on Low for 7 hours.
2. Divide the mix between plates, add the couscous on the side, sprinkle the sage on top, and serve.

Nutrition: Calories: 272 | Fats: 14.5 g | Carbs: 16.3g | Protein: 14.3 g

Ingredients:

- 2 pounds pork loin boneless and sliced
- ¾ cup veggie stock
- 2 tablespoons olive oil
- ½ tablespoon chili powder
- 2 teaspoon sage, dried
- ½ tablespoon garlic powder
- Salt and black pepper to taste
- 2 cups couscous, cooked

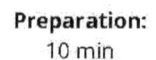

Pork Fajitas

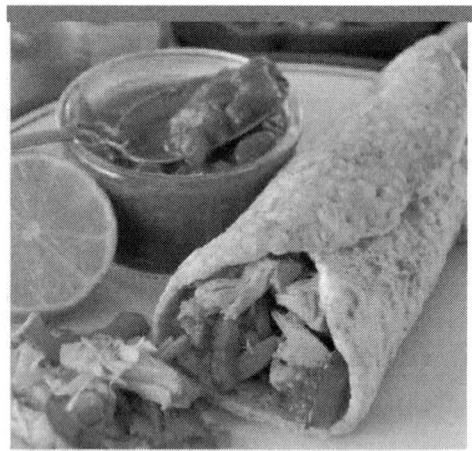

Preparation: 10 min
Cooking: 20 min
Servings: 4

Directions:

1. Start by mixing the oregano, garlic, vinegar, cumin, hot sauce, and pineapple juice in a bowl.
2. Place the pork in this marinade and mix well to coat them, then refrigerate for 15 minutes.
3. Meanwhile, preheat your oven to 325°F.
4. Wrap the tortillas in foil and heat them in the oven for 2-3 minutes.
5. Now, heat a suitable griddle on medium fire and add pork strips, green peppers, oil, and onion.
6. Cook for 5 minutes until pork is done.
7. Serve warm in warmed tortillas.

Nutrition: Calories:406 | Protein: 26 g | Carbs: 34 g | Fat: 18 g

Ingredients:

- 1 green bell pepper, julienned
- 1 medium onion, julienned
- 2 garlic cloves, minced
- 1 lb. lean, boneless pork cut into strips
- 1 teaspoon dried oregano
- ½ teaspoons cumin
- 2 tablespoons pineapple juice
- 2 tablespoons vinegar
- ¼ teaspoon hot pepper sauce
- 1 tablespoon olive oil
- 4 flour tortillas, 8" size

Apple Spice Pork Chops

Ingredients:
- 1 pound pork chops
- 2 tablespoons olive oil
- ¼ cup brown sugar
- ¼ teaspoon salt (or exclude to reduce sodium)
- ¼ teaspoon pepper
- ¼ teaspoon nutmeg
- ¼ teaspoon cinnamon
- 2 medium tart apples

Preparation: 10 min **Cooking:** 35 min **Servings:** 4

Directions:
1. Preheat the oven to broil.
2. Peel and slice the apples.
3. Broil the pork chops in the oven for about 4 to 5 minutes on both sides.
4. In a skillet, add the oil, stirring in the brown sugar, salt, nutmeg, cinnamon, pepper, and apples.
5. Cover and cook until the apples become tender and the sauce starts to thicken.
6. Spoon out the sauce over the cooked chops and serve.

Tips:
- Marinate the pork chops in the apple juice, pepper, and chopped garlic for additional flavor.
- A hot skillet can also be used to cook the pork chops instead of broiling. To do this, brush the chops with oil and cook for about 5 minutes on each side.

Nutrition: Calories: 306 | Protein: 22 g | Carbs: 21 g | Fats: 16 g |

Beef Burritos

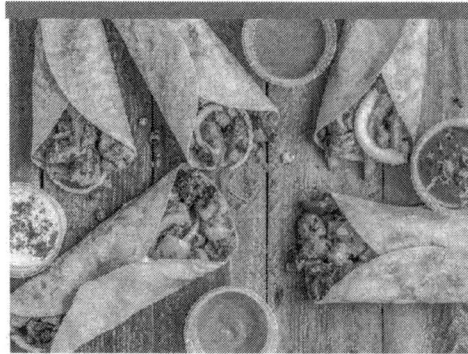

Preparation: 25 min **Cooking:** 20 min **Servings:** 6

Ingredients:
- ¼ cup onion
- ¼ cup green pepper
- 1-pound lean ground beef
- ¼ cup tomato puree
- ¼ teaspoon black pepper
- ¼ teaspoon ground cumin
- 6 burrito-size flour tortillas

Directions:
1. Chop the onion and green pepper.
2. Brown the ground beef in a medium skillet and drain on paper towels.
3. Grease the skillet with non-stick cooking spray, then add the onion and green pepper. Cook for about 3 to 5 minutes or until the vegetables become softened.
4. Add the beef, tomato puree, cumin, and black pepper to the onion and pepper mixture. Mix properly and cook over low heat for about 3 to 5 minutes.
5. Divide the beef mixture among the tortillas and roll the tortilla over burrito style. Make sure both ends are first folded so that the mixture doesn't fall off.

Nutrition: Calories: 265 | Protein: 15 g | Carbs: 31 g | Fats: 9 g

Chapter 7

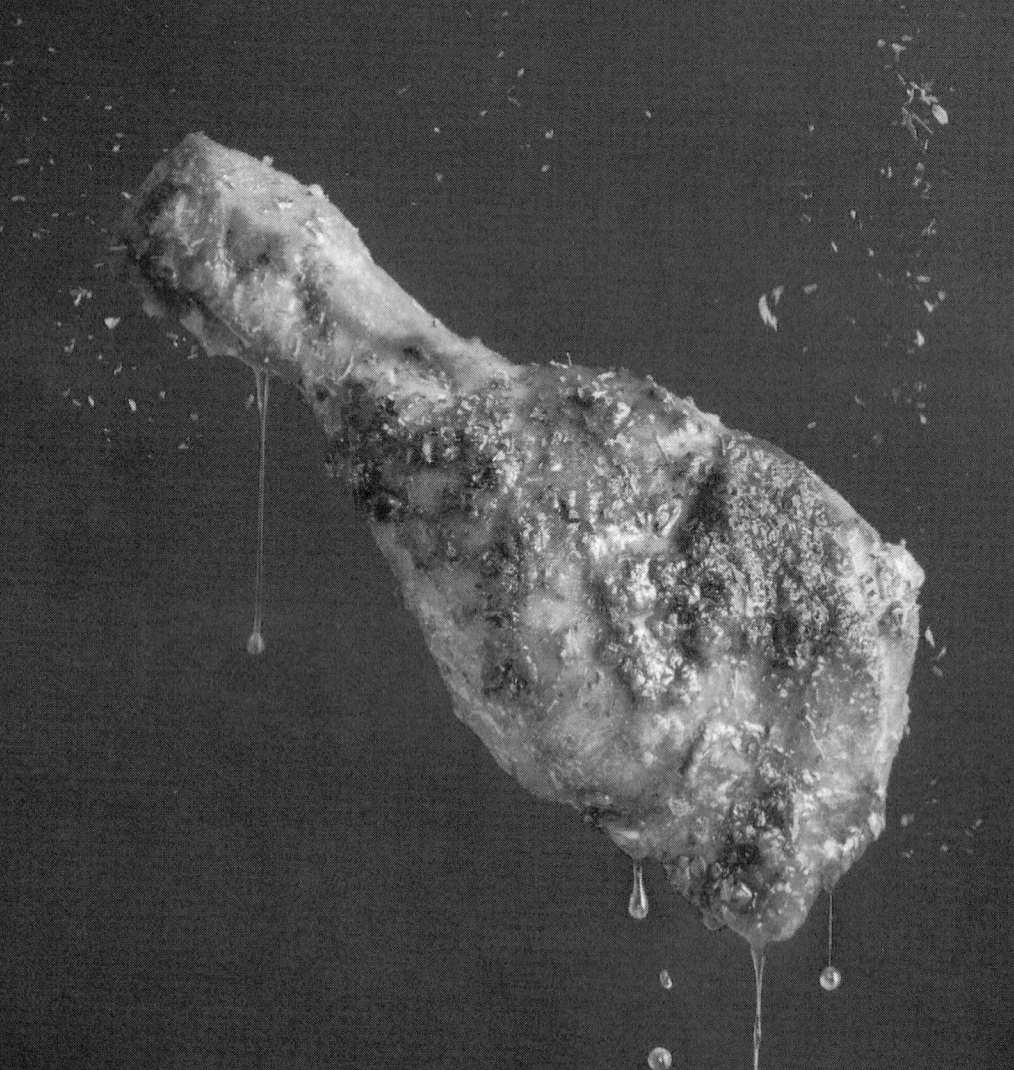

Poultry

Oven Roasted Garlic Chicken Thigh

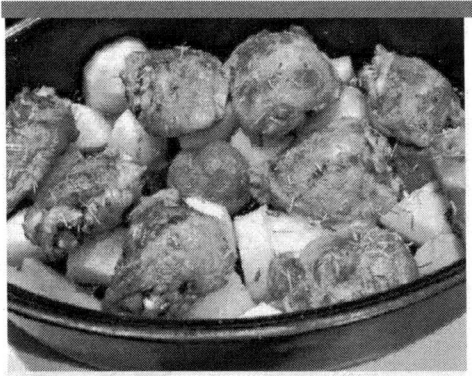

Preparation: 10 min

Cooking: 55 min

Servings: 2

Directions:

1. Season the chicken with kosher salt and black pepper.
2. Heat olive oil on a cast-iron skillet over a medium-high fire.
3. Sear the chicken on both sides.
4. Add the remaining ingredients except for basil and stir well.
5. Remove heat and place cast iron skillet in the oven.
6. Bake for 45 minutes at 400°F until the internal temperature reaches 165°F.
7. Serve and enjoy!

Nutrition: Calories: 500 | Fats: 23 g | Carbs: 37 g | Protein: 35 g

Ingredients:

- 8 chicken thighs
- Salt and pepper as needed
- 1 tablespoon extra-virgin olive oil
- 6 cloves garlic, peeled and crushed
- 1 jar (10 ounces) roasted red peppers, drained and chopped
- 1 ½ pounds potatoes, diced
- 2 cups cherry tomatoes, halved
- 1/3 cup capers, sliced
- 1 teaspoon dried Italian seasoning
- 1 tablespoon fresh basil

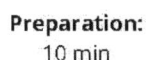

Grilled Harissa Chicken

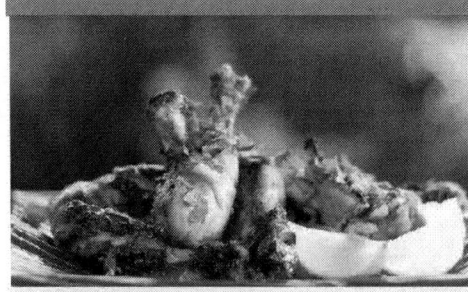

Preparation: 20 min

Cooking: 15 min

Servings: 2

Directions:

1. Get a large bowl. Season your chicken with kosher salt on all sides; then add onions, garlic, lemon juice, and harissa paste to the bowl.
2. Add about 3 tablespoons of olive oil to the mixture. Heat a grill to 459°F (an indoor or outdoor grill works just fine), then oil the grates.
3. Grill each side of the chicken for about 7 minutes. Its temperature should register 165°F on a thermometer, and it should be fully cooked by then.

Nutrition: Calories: 142.5 | Fats: 4.7 g | Carbs: 1.7 g | Protein: 22.1 g

Ingredients:

- 1 lemon, juiced
- ½ sliced red onion
- 1 ½ teaspoon coriander
- 1 ½ teaspoon smoked paprika
- 1 teaspoon cumin
- 2 teaspoons cayenne
- 3 tablespoon olive oil
- 1 ½ teaspoon Black pepper
- Kosher salt
- 5 ounces thawed and drained frozen spinach
- 8 boneless chickens

Italian Chicken Meatballs

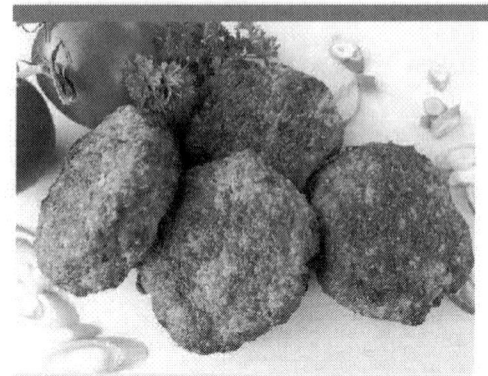

Preparation: 20 min
Cooking: 32 min
Servings: 20

Ingredients:
- 3 tomatoes
- Kosher salt
- ½ cup freshly chopped parsley
- 1 teaspoon dry oregano
- Kosher salt
- ½ teaspoon fresh thyme
- ¼ teaspoon sweet paprika
- 1 red onion
- 1 lb. ground chicken
- ½ minced garlic cloves
- Black pepper
- 1 raw egg
- ¼ cup freshly grated parmesan cheese
- Extra virgin olive oil

Directions:
1. Heat the oven to 375°F and get a cooking pan. Coat with extra virgin olive oil and set aside.
2. Get a large bowl and mix your tomatoes with kosher salt and thinly chopped onions.
3. Add half of your fresh thyme and sprinkle a little extra virgin olive oil on it again.
4. Transfer this to your cooking pan and use a spoon to spread. Add ground chicken to the mixing bowl you recently used, and add egg, parmesan cheese, and oregano.
5. Include paprika, garlic, the other half of thyme, chopped parsley, and black pepper.
6. Sprinkle a little extra virgin olive oil on it, and mix until the meatball mixture is combined. Form about 1 ½ inch chicken meatballs with the mixture and cut it all to this size.
7. Get another cooking pan and arrange these meatballs in it. Add tomatoes and onions, and blend them with the meatballs. Bake in your preheated oven for about 30 minutes.
8. Your meatballs should turn golden brown, you can make them more colorful by removing them and coating them with extra virgin olive oil before you continue baking.
9. But that is not necessary. A couple of minutes after this, your meatballs cam is served.
10. No surprises, your tomatoes are fast falling.

Nutrition: Calories: 79 | Fiber: 0.92 g | Carbs: 4.1 g | Protein: 17.8 g

Classic Chicken Cooking With Tomatoes & Tapenade

Ingredients:
- 4-5 ounces chicken breasts, boneless and skinless
- ¼ teaspoon salt (divided)
- 3 tablespoons fresh basil leaves, chopped (divided)
- 1 tablespoon olive oil
- 1 ½ cups cherry tomatoes, halved
- ¼ cup olive tapenade

Preparation: 25 min
Cooking: 25 min
Servings: 2

Directions:
1. Arrange the chicken on a sheet of glassine or waxed paper. Sprinkle half of the salt and a third of the basil evenly over the chicken.
2. Press lightly, and flip over the chicken pieces. Sprinkle the remaining salt and another third of the basil. Cover the seasoned chicken with another sheet of waxed paper.
3. By using a meat mallet or rolling pin, pound the chicken to a half-inch thickness.
4. Heat the olive oil in a 12-inch skillet placed over a medium-high fire. Add the pounded chicken breasts.
5. Cook for 6 minutes on each side until the chicken turns golden brown with no traces of pink in the middle. Transfer the browned chicken breasts to a platter, and cover them to keep them warm.
6. In the same skillet, add the olive tapenade and tomatoes. Cook for 3 minutes until the tomatoes just begin to be tender.
7. To serve, pour the tomato-tapenade mixture over the cooked chicken breasts, and top with the remaining basil.

Nutrition: Calories: 190 | Fats: 7 g | Carbs: 6 g | Protein: 26 g

Grilled Grapes & Chicken Chunks

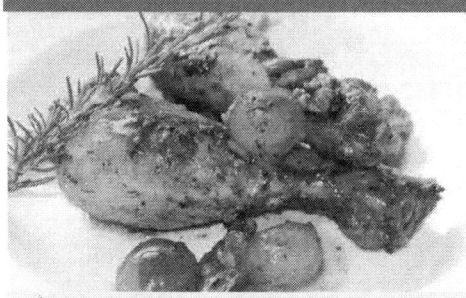

Preparation: 15 min
Cooking: 30 min
Servings: 2

Ingredients:

- 2 garlic cloves, minced
- ¼ cup extra-virgin olive oil
- 1 tablespoon rosemary, minced
- 1 tablespoon oregano, minced
- 1 teaspoon lemon zest
- ½ teaspoon red chili flakes, crushed
- 1 lb. chicken breast, boneless and skinless
- 1 ¾ cups green grapes, seedless and rinsed
- ½ teaspoon salt
- 1 tablespoon lemon juice

Directions:

1. Combine and mix all the marinade ingredients in a small mixing bowl. Mix well until fully combined. Set aside.
2. Cut the chicken breast into ¾-inch cubes. Alternately, thread the chicken and grapes onto 12 skewers. Place the skewers in a large baking dish to hold them for marinating.
3. Pour the marinade over the skewers, coating them thoroughly. Marinate for 4 to 24 hours.
4. Remove the skewers from the marinade and allow dripping off any excess oil. Sprinkle over with salt.
5. Grill the chicken and grape skewers for 3 minutes on each side until cooked through.
6. To serve, arrange the skewers on a serving platter and drizzle them with lemon juice and olive oil.

Nutrition: Calories: 290 | Fats: 12 g | Carbs: 14 g | Protein: 28 g

Turkish Turkey Mini Meatloaves

Ingredients:

- 1 lb. ground turkey breast
- 1 egg
- ¼ cup whole-wheat breadcrumbs, crushed
- ¼ cup feta cheese, plus more for topping
- ¼ cup Kalamata olives, halved
- ¼ cup fresh parsley, chopped
- ¼ cup red onion, minced
- ¼ cup + 2 tablespoons hummus
- 2 garlic cloves, minced
- ½ teaspoon dried basil
- ¼ teaspoon dried oregano
- ½ small cucumber, peeled, seeded, and chopped
- 1 large tomato, chopped
- 3 tablespoons fresh basil, chopped
- ½ lemon, juice
- 1 teaspoon extra-virgin olive oil
- Salt and pepper

Preparation: 15 min
Cooking: 20 min
Servings: 2

Directions:

1. Preheat your oven to 425°F.
2. Line a 5x9" baking sheet with foil, and spray the surfaces with non-stick grease. Set aside.
3. Except for the ¼ cup hummus, combine and mix all the turkey meatloaf ingredients in a large mixing bowl. Mix well until fully combined.
4. Divide the mixture equally into 4 portions. Form the portions into loaves. Spread a tablespoon of the remaining hummus on each meatloaf. Place the loaves on the greased baking sheet.
5. Bake for 20 minutes until the loaves no longer appear pink in the center. (Ensure the meatloaf cooks through by inserting a meat thermometer and the reading reaches 165°F)
6. Combine and mix all the topping ingredients in a small mixing bowl. Mix well until fully combined.
7. To serve, spoon the topping over the cooked meatloaves.

Nutrition: Calories: 220 | Fats: 12 g | Carbs: 14 g | Protein: 26 g

Lemon Caper Chicken

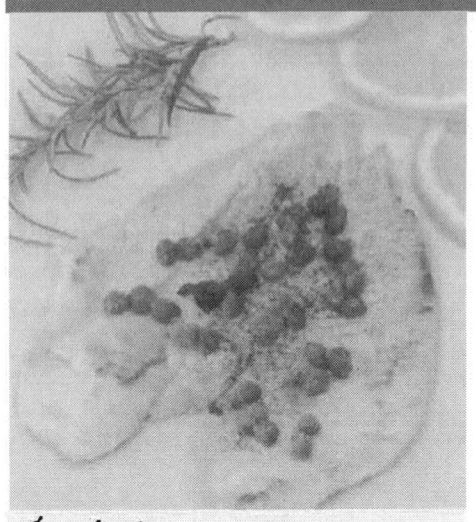

Preparation: 10 min

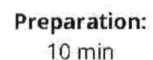

Cooking: 15 min

Servings: 2

Directions:

1. Take a large skillet, place it on your stove, and add olive oil. Turn the heat to medium and allow it to warm up.
2. As the oil heats, season your chicken breast with the oregano, basil, and black pepper on each side.
3. Place your chicken breast into the hot skillet and cook on each side for five minutes.
4. Transfer the chicken from the skillet to your dinner plate. Top with capers and serve with a few lemon wedges.

Nutrition: Calories: 282 | Carbs: 3.4 g | Protein: 26.6 g | Fats: 8.2 g

Ingredients:

- 2 tablespoon virgin olive oil
- 2 chicken breasts (boneless, skinless, cut in half, pound to ¾ an inch thick)
- ¼ cup capers
- 2 lemons (wedges)
- 1 teaspoon oregano
- 1 teaspoon basil
- ½ teaspoon black pepper

Herb Roasted Chicken

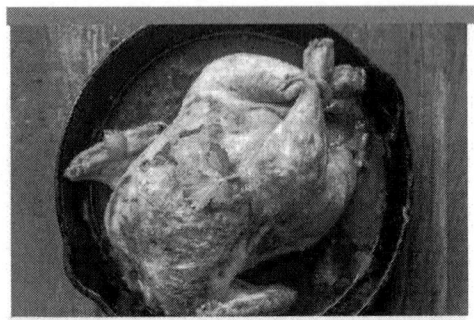

Preparation: 20 min

Cooking: 1 hr

Servings: 2

Directions:

1. Turn your oven to 450°F.
2. Take your whole chicken and pat it dry using paper towels. Then rub in the olive oil. Remove the leaves from one of the rosemary springs and scatter them over the chicken. Sprinkle the sea salt and black pepper over the top. Place the other whole sprig of rosemary into the cavity of the chicken. Then add in the garlic cloves and lemon halves.
3. Place the chicken into a roasting pan and then into the oven. Allow the chicken to bake for 1 hour, then check that the internal temperature should be at least 165°F. If the chicken begins to brown too much, cover it with foil and return it to the oven to finish cooking.
4. When the chicken has cooked to the appropriate temperature, remove it from the oven. Let it rest for at least 20 minutes before carving.
5. Serve with a large side of roasted or steamed vegetables or your favorite salad.

Nutrition: Calories: 309 | Carbs: 1.5 g | Protein: 27.2 g | Fats: 16.3 g

Ingredients:

- 1 tablespoon virgin olive oil
- 1 whole chicken
- 2 rosemary springs
- 3 garlic cloves (peeled)
- 1 lemon (cut in half)
- 1 teaspoon sea salt
- 1 teaspoon black pepper

Grilled Chicken Breasts

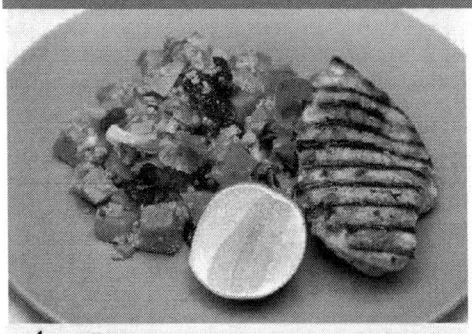

Preparation: 10 min

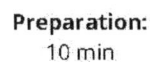

Cooking: 15 min

Servings: 2

Ingredients:

- 4 boneless skinless chicken breasts
- 3 tablespoons lemon juice
- 3 tablespoons olive oil
- 3 tablespoons chopped fresh parsley
- 3 minced garlic cloves
- 1 teaspoon paprika
- ½ teaspoon dried oregano
- Salt and pepper to taste

Directions:

1. In a large Ziploc bag, mix well oregano, paprika, garlic, parsley, olive oil, and lemon juice.
2. Pierce chicken with a knife several times and sprinkle with salt and pepper.
3. Add chicken to the bag and marinate in the fridge for 20 minutes or up to two days.
4. Remove chicken from the bag and grill for 5 minutes per side on a 350F preheated grill.
5. When cooked, transfer to a plate for 5 minutes before slicing.
6. Serve and enjoy with a side of rice or salad

Nutrition: Calories: 238 | Protein: 24 g | Carbs: 2 g | Fats: 14 g

Turkey Meatballs

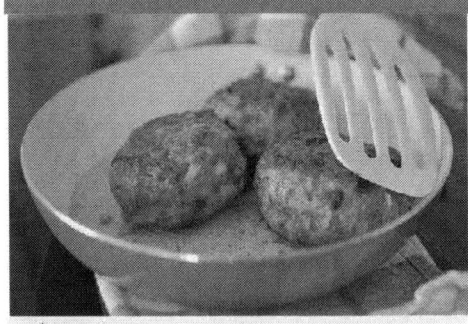

Preparation: 10 min

Cooking: 25 min

Servings: 2

Ingredients:

- ¼ diced yellow onion
- 14 ounces diced artichoke hearts
- 1 lb ground turkey
- 1 teaspoon dried parsley
- 1 teaspoon oil
- 4 tablespoons chopped basil
- Pepper and salt to taste

Directions:

1. Grease the baking sheet and preheat the oven to 350°F.
2. On medium heat, place a nonstick medium saucepan. Sauté artichoke hearts and diced onions for 5 minutes or until onions are soft.
3. Meanwhile, in a big bowl, mix parsley, basil, and ground turkey with your hands. Season to taste.
4. Once the onion mixture has cooled, add it to the bowl and mix thoroughly.
5. With an ice cream scooper, scoop ground turkey and form balls.
6. Place on a prepared cooking sheet, pop in the oven, and bake until cooked, around 15-20 minutes.
7. Remove from pan, serve and enjoy.

Nutrition: Calories: 283 | Protein: 12 g | Carbs: 30 g | Fats: 12 g

Chicken Marsala

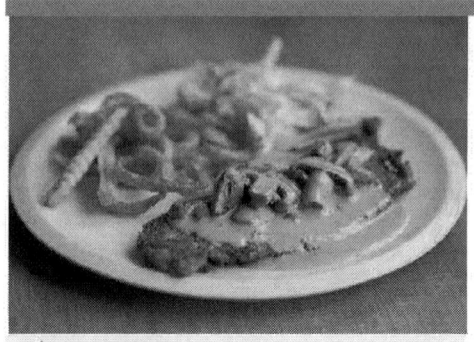

Preparation: 10 min

Cooking: 45 min

Servings: 2

Ingredients:

- 2 tablespoons olive oil
- 4 skinless, boneless chicken breast cutlets
- ¾ tablespoons black pepper, divided
- ½ teaspoon kosher salt, divided
- 8 ounces mushrooms, sliced
- 4 thyme sprigs
- 0.2 quarts unsalted chicken stock
- 2 Quarts marsala wine
- A handful of Fresh thyme, chopped

Directions:

1. Heat oil in a pan and fry the chicken for 4-5 minutes per side. Remove chicken from the pan and set it aside.
2. In the same pan, add thyme, mushrooms, salt, and pepper; stir fry for 1-2 minutes.
3. Add Marsala wine, chicken broth, and cooked chicken. Let simmer for 10-12 minutes on low heat.
4. Add to a serving dish.
5. Enjoy.

Nutrition: Calories: 206 | Fats: 12 g | Carbs: 3 g | Protein: 18 g

Lean and Green Chicken Pesto Pasta

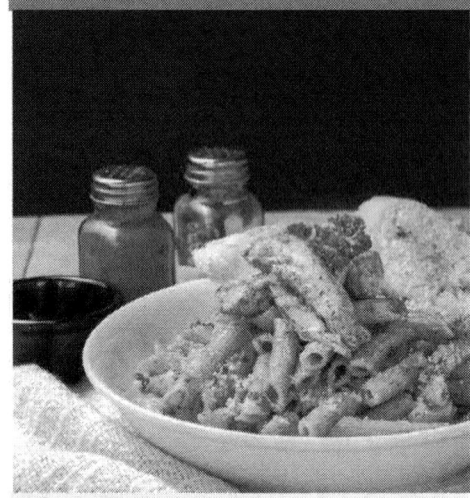

Preparation: 5 min

Cooking: 15 min

Servings: 1

Ingredients:

- 3 cups raw kale leaves
- 2 tablespoons olive oil
- 2 cups fresh basil
- ¼ teaspoon salt
- 3 tablespoons lemon juice
- 3 garlic cloves
- 2 cups cooked chicken breast
- 1 cup baby spinach
- 6 ounces uncooked pasta
- 3 ounces diced fresh mozzarella
- Basil leaves or red pepper flakes to garnish

Directions:

1. Start by making the pesto, add the kale, lemon juice, basil, garlic cloves, olive oil, and salt to a blender and blend until it's smooth.
2. Add salt and pepper to taste.
3. Cook the pasta and strain off the water. Reserve ¼ cup of the liquid.
4. Get a bowl and mix the cooked pasta, pesto, diced chicken, spinach, mozzarella, and the reserved pasta liquid.
5. Sprinkle the mixture with additional chopped basil or red paper flakes (optional).
6. Now your salad is ready. You may serve it warm or chilled. Also, it can be taken as a salad mix-in or as a side dish. Leftovers should be stored in the refrigerator inside an air-tight container for 3-5 days.

Nutrition: Calories: 244 | Protein: 20.5 g | Carbs: 22.5 g | Fats: 10 g

Chicken Stuffed Peppers

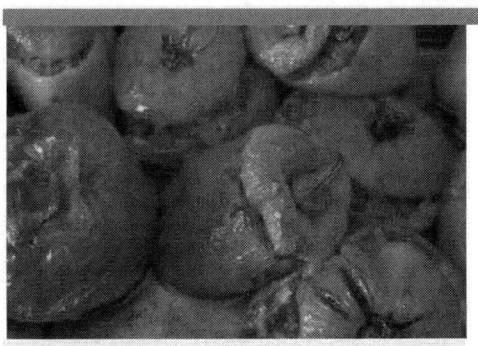

Preparation: 10 min
Cooking: 0 min
Servings: 6

Ingredients:
- 1 cup Greek yogurt
- 2 tablespoons mustard
- Salt and black pepper to taste
- 1 pound rotisserie chicken meat, cubed
- 4 celery stalks, chopped
- 2 tablespoons balsamic vinegar
- 1 bunch scallions, sliced
- ¼ cup parsley, chopped
- 1 cucumber, sliced
- 3 red bell peppers, halved and deseeded
- 1-pint cherry tomatoes, quartered

Directions:
1. In a bowl, mix the chicken with the celery and the rest of the ingredients except the bell peppers and toss well.
2. Stuff the peppers halves with the chicken mix and serve for lunch.

Nutrition: Calories: 266 | Fats: 12.2 | Carbs: 15.7 | Protein: 3.7

Turkey Fritters and Sauce

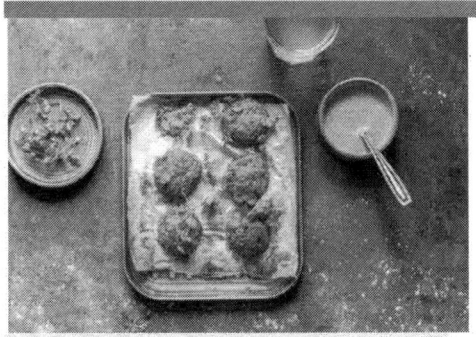

Preparation: 10 min
Cooking: 30 min
Servings: 3

Ingredients:
- 2 garlic cloves, minced
- 1 egg
- 1 red onion, chopped
- 1 tablespoon olive oil
- ¼ teaspoon red pepper flakes
- 1 pound turkey meat, ground
- ½ teaspoon oregano, dried
- Cooking spray

For the sauce:
- 1 cup Greek yogurt
- 1 cucumber, chopped
- 1 tablespoon olive oil
- ¼ teaspoon garlic powder
- 2 tablespoons lemon juice
- ¼ cup parsley, chopped

Directions:
1. Heat a pan with 1 tablespoon oil over medium fire. Add the onion and the garlic, sauté for 5 minutes, cool down and transfer to a bowl.
2. Add the meat, turkey, oregano, and pepper flakes. Stir and shape medium fritters out of this mix.
3. Heat another pan greased with cooking spray over a medium-high fire. Add the turkey fritters and brown for 5 minutes on each side.
4. Introduce the pan to the oven and bake the fritters at 375°F for 15 minutes more.
5. Meanwhile, in a bowl, mix the yogurt with the cucumber, oil, garlic powder, lemon juice, and parsley, and whisk well.
6. Divide the fritters between plates, spread the sauce, and serve for lunch.

Nutrition: Calories: 364 | Fats: 16.8 | Carbs: 26.8 | Protein: 23.4

Herbed Chicken Stew

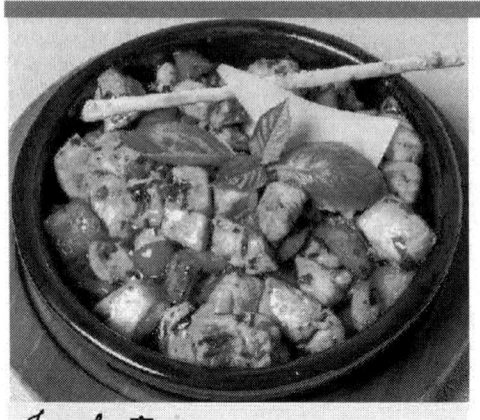

Preparation: 10 min
Cooking: 1 hr 30 min
Servings: 3

Directions:

1. Heat the oil in a skillet and place the chicken in the hot oil.
2. Cook on each side until golden brown. Then add the shallots, garlic, and pesto sauce.
3. Cook for 2 more minutes, then add the rest of the ingredients and half a cup of water.
4. Season with salt and pepper and continue cooking on low heat, covered with a lid, for 30 minutes.
5. Serve the stew warm or fresh.

Nutrition: Calories: 357 | Fats: 19.6 g | Protein: 41.4 g | Carbs: 2.0 g

Ingredients:

- 3 tablespoons olive oil
- 6 chicken legs
- 2 shallots, chopped
- 4 garlic cloves, minced
- 2 tablespoons pesto sauce
- ½ cup chopped cilantro
- ½ cup chopped parsley
- 2 tablespoons lemon juice
- 4 tablespoons vegetable stock
- Salt and pepper to taste

Grilled Chicken

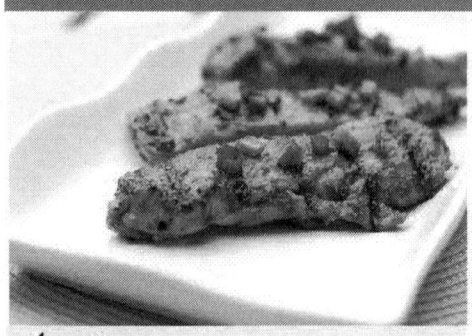

Preparation: 15 min
Cooking: 15 min
Servings: 4

Directions:

1. Add lemon juice, oregano, paprika, garlic, parsley, and olive oil to a large zip-lock bag. Season chicken with pepper and salt and add to the bag. Seal the bag, shake well to coat the chicken, and marinate for 20 minutes.
2. Remove chicken from the marinade and grill over medium-high heat for 5-6 minutes on each side. Serve and enjoy.

Nutrition: Calories: 512 | Fats: 36.5 g | Protein: 43.1 g | Carbs: 3 g |

Ingredients:

- 4 chicken breasts, skinless and boneless
- 1 ½ teaspoon dried oregano
- 1 teaspoon paprika
- 5 garlic cloves, minced
- ½ cup fresh parsley, minced
- ½ cup olive oil
- ½ cup fresh lemon juice
- Pepper
- Salt

Turkey With Leeks and Radishes

Ingredients:
- 1-pound turkey breast, skinless, boneless, and cubed
- 1 leek, sliced
- 1 cup radishes, sliced
- 1 red onion, chopped
- 1 tablespoon olive oil
- A pinch salt and black pepper
- 1 cup chicken stock
- ½ teaspoon sweet paprika
- ½ teaspoon coriander, ground
- 1 tablespoon cilantro, chopped

Preparation: 10 min
Cooking: 6 hrs
Servings: 2

Directions:
1. In your slow cooker, combine the turkey with the leek, radishes, onion, and the other ingredients; toss, put the lid on and cook on Low for 6 hours.
2. Divide everything between plates and serve.

Nutrition: Calories: 226 | Fat: 9 g | Carbs: 6 g | Protein: 28 g

Turkey and Cranberry Sauce

Ingredients:
- 1 cup chicken stock
- 2 tablespoons avocado oil
- ½ cup cranberry sauce
- 1 big turkey breast, skinless, boneless, and sliced
- 1 yellow onion, roughly chopped
- Salt and black pepper to taste

Preparation: 10 min
Cooking: 50 min
Servings: 3

Directions:
1. Heat a pan with the avocado oil over medium-high fire. Add the onion and sauté for 5 minutes.
2. Add the turkey and brown for 5 minutes more.
3. Add the rest of the ingredients, toss, introduce in the oven at 350°F and cook for 40 minutes.
4. Serve with cranberry sauce.

Nutrition: Calories: 382 | Fats: 12.6 g | Carbs: 26.6g | Protein: 17.6 g

Coconut Chicken

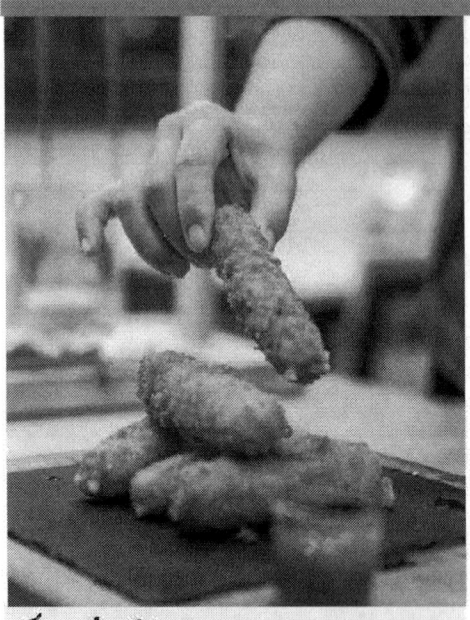

Preparation: 10 min

Cooking: 5 min

Servings: 3

Directions:

1. Cut the chicken fillet into small pieces (nuggets).
2. Then crack the egg in the bowl and whisk it.
3. Mix the egg and sparkling water.
4. Add Greek seasoning and stir gently.
5. Dip the chicken nuggets in the egg mixture and then coat in the coconut flakes.
6. Melt the coconut oil in the skillet and heat it until it is shimmering.
7. Then add prepared chicken nuggets.
8. Roast them for 1 minute from each or until they are light brown.
9. Dry the cooked chicken nuggets with the help of a paper towel and transfer them to the serving plates.

Nutrition: Calories: 141 | Fats: 8.9g | Carbs: 1g | Protein: 13.9 g

Ingredients:

- 6 ounces chicken fillet
- ¼ cup sparkling water
- 1 egg
- 3 tablespoons coconut flakes
- 1 tablespoon coconut oil
- 1 teaspoon Greek Seasoning

Ginger Chicken Drumsticks

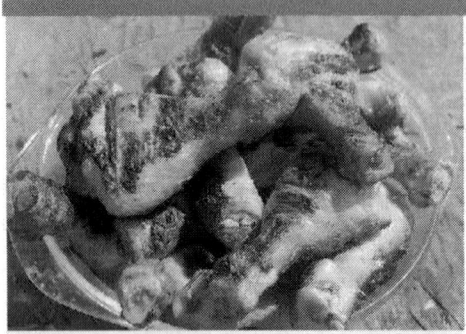

Preparation: 10 min

Cooking: 30 min

Servings: 4

Directions:

1. Mix grated apple, curry paste, milk, chili flakes, and minced garlic.
2. Put coconut oil in the skillet and melt it.
3. Add apple mixture and stir well.
4. Then add chicken drumsticks and mix up well.
5. Roast the chicken for 2 minutes from each side.
6. Then preheat the oven to 360°F.
7. Place the skillet with chicken drumsticks in the oven and bake for 25 minutes.

Nutrition: Calories: 150 | Fats: 6.4 g| Carbs: 9.7g | Protein: 13.5 g

Ingredients:

- 4 chicken drumsticks
- 1 apple, grated
- 1 tablespoon curry paste
- 4 tablespoons milk
- 1 teaspoon coconut oil
- 1 teaspoon chili flakes
- ½ teaspoon minced ginger

Pomegranate Chicken

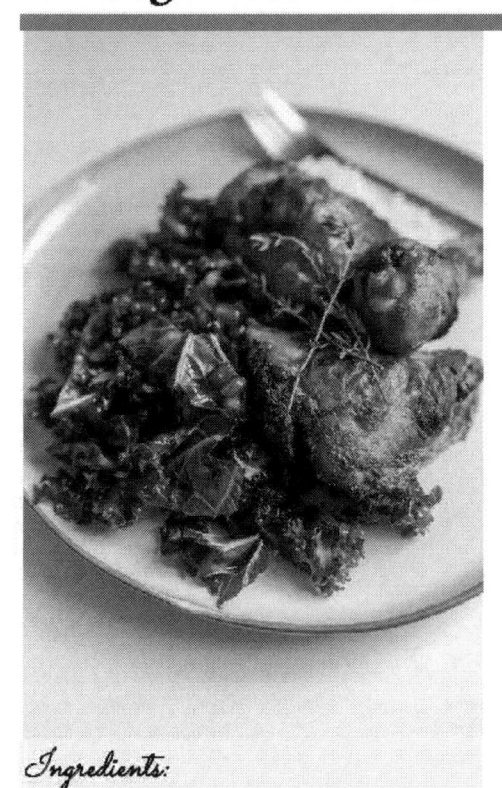

Preparation: 10 min
Cooking: 30 min
Servings: 6

Directions:

1. Rub the chicken breast with za'atar seasoning, salt, olive oil, and pomegranate juice.
2. Marinate the chicken for 15 minutes and transfer it to the skillet.
3. Roast the chicken for 15 minutes over medium heat.
4. Then flip the chicken to another side and cook for 10 minutes more.
5. Slice the chicken and place it on the serving plates.

Nutrition: Calories: 107 | Fats: 4.2 g| Carbs: 0.2 g| Protein: 16.1 g

Ingredients:

- 1-pound 4 chicken drumsticks
- 1 tablespoon za'atar
- ½ teaspoon salt
- 1 tablespoon pomegranate juice
- 1 tablespoon olive oil

Lemon Chicken Mix

Ingredients:

- 8 ounces chicken breast, skinless, boneless
- 1 teaspoon Cajun seasoning
- 1 teaspoon balsamic vinegar
- 1 teaspoon olive oil
- 1 teaspoon lemon juice

Preparation: 10 min
Cooking: 10 min
Servings: 3

Directions:

1. Cut the chicken breast into halves and sprinkle with Cajun seasoning.
2. Then sprinkle the poultry with olive oil and lemon juice.
3. Next, sprinkle the chicken breast with balsamic vinegar.
4. Preheat the grill to 385°F.
5. Grill the chicken breast halves for 5 minutes from each side.
6. Slice the Cajun chicken and place it on the serving plate.

Nutrition: Calories: 150 | Fats: 5.2g | Carbs: 0.1 g| Protein: 24.1 g

Cardamom Chicken and Apricot Sauce

Ingredients:
- ½ lemon, juiced
- Zest of ½ lemon, grated
- 2 teaspoons cardamom, ground
- Salt and black pepper to taste
- 2 chicken breasts, skinless, boneless, and halved
- 2 tablespoons olive oil
- 2 spring onions, chopped
- 2 tablespoons tomato paste
- 2 garlic cloves, minced
- 1 cup apricot juice
- ½ cup chicken stock
- ¼ cup cilantro, chopped

Preparation: 10 min
Cooking: 7 min
Servings: 3

Directions:
1. In your slow cooker, combine the chicken with the lemon juice, lemon zest, and the other ingredients except for the cilantro. Toss, put the lid on, and cook on Low for 7 hours.
2. Divide the mix between plates, sprinkle the cilantro on top, and serve.

Nutrition: Calories: 323 | Fats: 12 g | Carbs: 23.8 g | Protein: 16.4 g

Chicken and Spinach Cakes

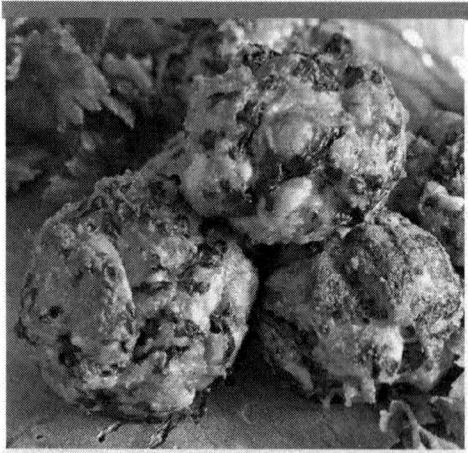

Preparation: 10 min
Cooking: 15 min
Servings: 3

Directions:
1. In the mixing bowl, mix ground chicken, blended spinach, minced garlic, salt, ground bell pepper, egg, and ground black pepper.
2. When the chicken mixture is smooth, make 4 burgers from it and coat them in Panko breadcrumbs.
3. Place the burgers in the non-sticky baking dish or line the baking tray with baking paper.
4. Bake the burgers for 15 minutes at 365°F.
5. Flip the chicken burgers on another side after 7 minutes of cooking.
6. Serve warm and enjoy.

Nutrition: Calories: 171 | Fats: 5.7g | Carbs: 10.5g | Protein: 19.4 g

Ingredients:
- 8 ounces ground chicken
- 1 cup fresh spinach, blended
- 1 teaspoon minced onion
- ½ teaspoon salt
- 1 red bell pepper, grinded
- 1 egg, beaten
- 1 teaspoon ground black pepper
- 4 tablespoons Panko breadcrumbs

Chicken and Parsley Sauce

Ingredients:
- 1 cup ground chicken
- 2 ounces Parmesan, grated
- 1 tablespoon olive oil
- 2 tablespoons fresh parsley, chopped
- 1 teaspoon chili pepper
- 1 teaspoon paprika
- ½ teaspoon dried oregano
- ¼ teaspoon garlic, minced
- ½ teaspoon dried thyme
- 1/3 cup crushed tomatoes

Preparation: 10 min
Cooking: 25 min
Servings: 3

Directions:
1. Heat olive oil in the skillet.
2. Add ground chicken and sprinkle it with chili pepper, paprika, dried oregano, dried thyme, and parsley. Mix up well.
3. Cook the chicken for 5 minutes and add crushed tomatoes. Mix up well.
4. Close the lid and simmer the chicken mixture for 10 minutes over low heat.
5. Then add grated Parmesan and mix up.
6. Cook chicken Bolognese for 5 minutes more over medium heat.
7. Serve warm.

Nutrition: Calories: 154 | Fats: 9.3g | Carbs: 3 g | Protein: 15.4 g

Chicken Marsala -day10: italian white bean soup

Ingredients:
- 1 big turkey breast, skinless, boneless, and roughly cubed
- 1 lemon, juiced
- 2 tablespoons avocado oil
- 1 red onion, chopped
- 2 tablespoons sage, chopped
- 1 garlic clove, minced
- 1 cup chicken stock

Preparation: 10 min
Cooking: 40 min
Servings: 3

Directions:
1. Heat a pan with the avocado oil over medium-high fire. Add the turkey and brown for 3 minutes on each side.
2. Add the rest of the ingredients to a simmer and cook over medium heat for 35 minutes.
3. Divide the mix between plates and serve with a side dish.

Nutrition: Calories: 382 | Fats: 12.6 g| Carbs: 16.6 | Protein: 33.2 g

Curry Chicken, Artichokes, and Olives

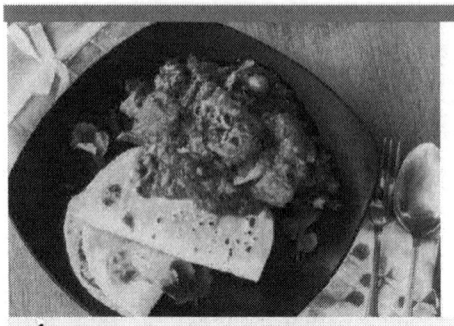

Preparation: 10 min
Cooking: 7 hrs
Servings: 3

Ingredients:

- 2 pounds chicken breasts, boneless, skinless, and cubed
- 12 ounces canned artichoke hearts, drained
- 1 cup chicken stock
- 1 red onion, chopped
- 1 tablespoon white wine vinegar
- 1 cup kalamata olives, pitted and chopped
- 1 tablespoon curry powder
- 2 teaspoons basil, dried
- Salt and black pepper to taste
- ¼ cup rosemary, chopped

Directions:

1. In your slow cooker, combine the chicken, artichokes, olives, and the rest of the ingredients; put the lid on, and cook on Low for 7 hours.
2. Divide the mix between plates and serve hot.

Nutrition: Calories: 275 | Fats: 11.9 g| Carbs: 19.7g | Protein: 18.7 g

Vegetable Ribbon Noodles with Chicken Breast Fillet

Ingredients:

- 250 g chicken breast fillet
- 1 medium-sized carrot
- 2 small zucchinis
- 2 medium-sized tomatoes
- 1 tablespoon tomato paste
- 50 ml vegetable broth
- 1 tablespoon olive oil
- ½ teaspoon paprika powder
- Salt and pepper

Preparation: 10 min
Cooking: 30 min
Servings: 2

Directions:

1. Cut the chicken breast fillet into bite-sized pieces. Heat the olive oil in a pan and add the paprika powder. Now sear the meat until it is completely cooked through. Season with a little salt and pepper.
2. In the meantime, wash and peel the carrots and cut lengthways into thin strips. Wash the zucchini and cut lengthways into thin strips.
3. Take the chicken out of the pan and sear the vegetable noodles in the remaining gravy for 3-4 minutes.
4. Wash the tomatoes and cut them into small pieces. Then add them to the vegetable noodles together with the tomato paste. Simmer for 3-4 minutes over medium heat. Season to taste with salt and pepper.
5. Add the chicken pieces and sear everything for 2-3 minutes.
6. Arrange on two plates and serve.

Nutrition: Calories: 300 | Total Fats: 17 g | Total Carbs: 34 g | Protein: 7 g

Zucchini and Mozzarella Casserole

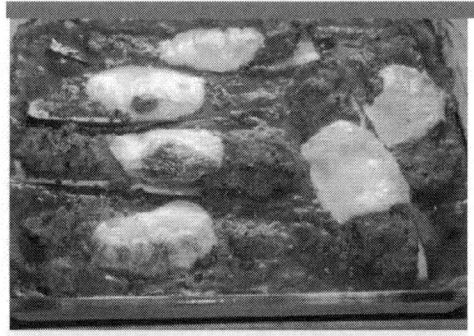

Preparation: 10 min
Cooking: 30 min
Servings: 2

Ingredients:
- 400 g ground poultry
- 125 g mozzarella
- 2 medium zucchinis
- 1 medium onion
- 1 garlic clove
- 1 tablespoon tomato paste
- 100 ml vegetable broth
- 2 teaspoons olive oil
- ½ teaspoon dried thyme
- ½ teaspoon dried oregano
- ½ teaspoon dried basil
- Salt and pepper

Directions:
1. Preheat the oven to 150°F top and bottom heat.
2. Wash the zucchini and cut it into thin slices.
3. Grease a baking dish with 1 teaspoon of olive oil and arrange some of the zucchini slices evenly in the dish.
4. Peel onions and cut them into fine pieces. Heat the remaining olive oil in a pan and fry the onion, garlic, and minced meat until it has a crumbly consistency. Then stir in the tomato paste, season with a little salt and pepper, and season with thyme, oregano, and basil.
5. Spread part of the minced meat mixture over the zucchini slices. Put another zucchini slice on top and distribute the remaining minced meat mixture on top.
6. Drain the mozzarella, cut it into slices, and spread it on the casserole.
7. Bake on the middle rack for 20-25 minutes.
8. Remove from the oven; let it cool down a little and serve.

Nutrition: Calories: 300 | Total Fats: 17 g | Total Carbs: 34 g | Protein: 27 g

Herby Chicken Meatloaf

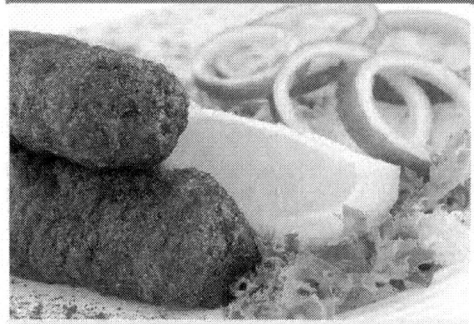

Preparation: 20 min
Cooking: 40 min
Servings: 6

Ingredients:
- 2 ½ lb. ground chicken
- 3 tablespoons flaxseed meal
- 2 large eggs
- 2 tablespoons olive oil
- 1 lemon, 1 tablespoon juice
- ¼ cup chopped parsley
- ¼ cup chopped oregano
- 4 garlic cloves, minced
- Lemon slices to garnish

Directions:
1. Preheat the oven to 400°F. In a bowl, combine ground chicken and flaxseed meal; set aside. In a small bowl, whisk the eggs with olive oil, lemon juice, parsley, oregano, and garlic.
2. Pour the mixture onto the chicken mixture and mix well. Spoon into a greased loaf pan and press to fit—bake for 40 minutes.
3. Remove the pan, drain the liquid, and let cool a bit. Slice, garnish with lemon slices, and serve.

Nutrition: Calories: 332 | Net Carbs: 1.3 g | Fats: 18 g | Protein: 35 g

Chapter 8

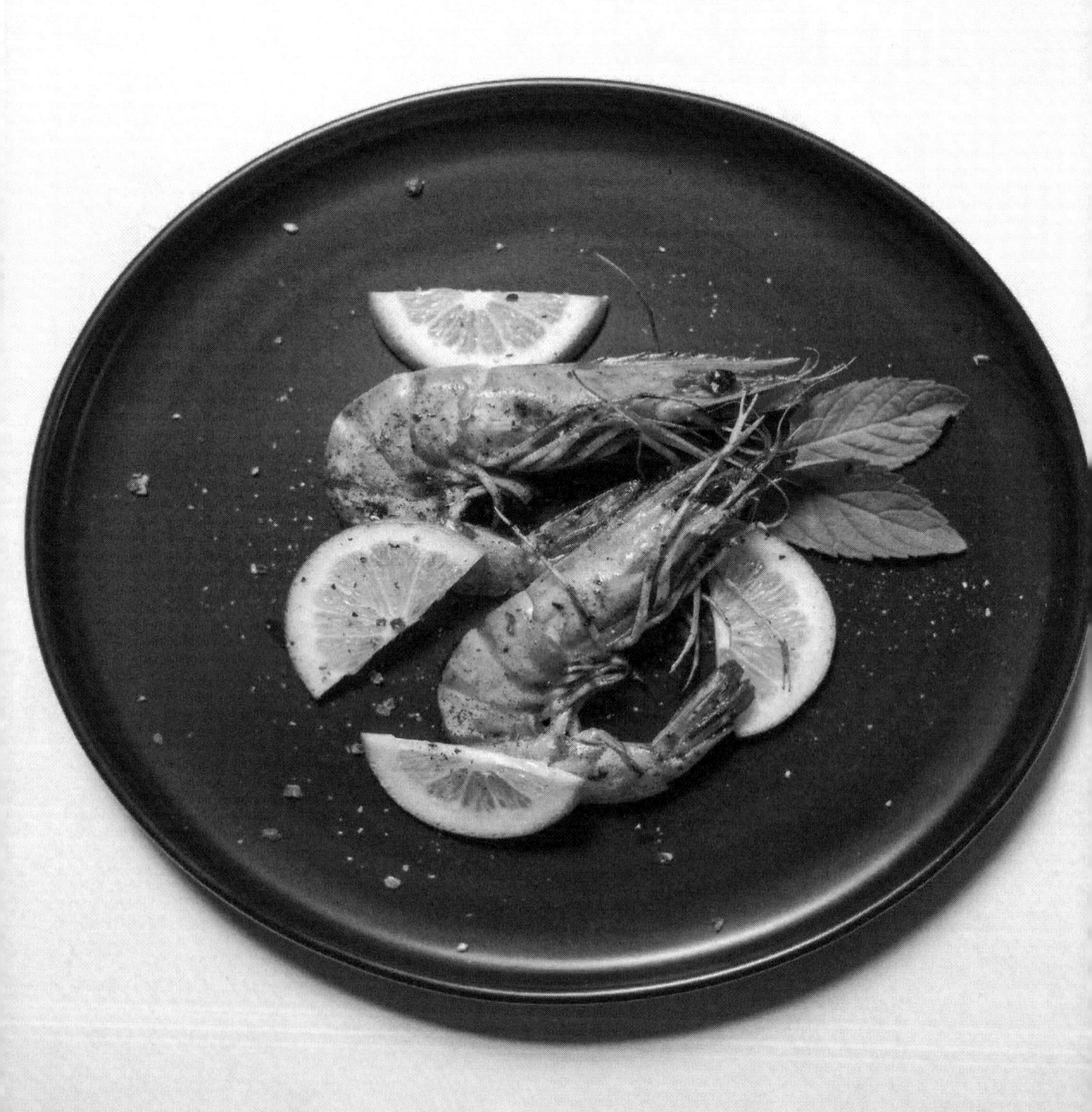

FISH & SEAFOOD

Tilapia with Avocado & Red Onion

Ingredients:
- 1 tablespoon olive oil
- 0.25 teaspoons sea salt
- 1 tablespoon fresh orange juice
- 4 (4-ounces) tilapia fillets (more rectangular than square)
- 0.25 cup red onion
- 1 sliced avocado

Also Needed: 9-inch pie plate

Preparation: 5 min | **Cooking:** 15 min | **Servings:** 4

Directions:
1. Combine the salt, juice, and oil to add to the pie dish. Work with one fillet at a time. Place it in the dish and turn to coat all sides.
2. Arrange the fillets in a wagon wheel-shaped formation. (Each fillet should be in the center of the dish with the other end draped over the edge.)
3. Place a tablespoon of the onion on top of each fillet and fold the end into the center. Cover the dish with plastic wrap, leaving one corner open to vent the steam.
4. Place in the microwave using the high heat setting for three minutes. It's done when the center can be easily flaked.
5. Top the fillets off with avocado and serve.

Nutrition: Calories: 200 | Protein: 22 g | Fats: 11 g

Herbed Roasted Cod

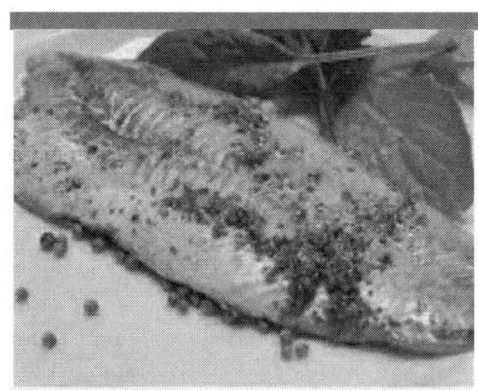

Ingredients:
- 4 cod fillets
- 4 parsley sprigs
- 2 cilantro sprigs
- 2 basil sprigs
- 1 lemon, sliced
- Salt and pepper to taste
- 2 tablespoons olive oil

Preparation: 10 min | **Cooking:** 45 min | **Servings:** 3

Directions:
1. Season the cod with salt and pepper.
2. Place the parsley, cilantro, basil, and lemon slices at the bottom of a deep-dish baking pan.
3. Place the cod over the herbs and cook in the preheated oven at 350°F for 15 minutes.
4. Serve the cod warm and fresh with your favorite side dish.

Nutrition: Calories: 192 | Fats:8.1 g | Protein: 28.6 g | Carbs: 0.1 g

Smoked Salmon and Watercress Salad

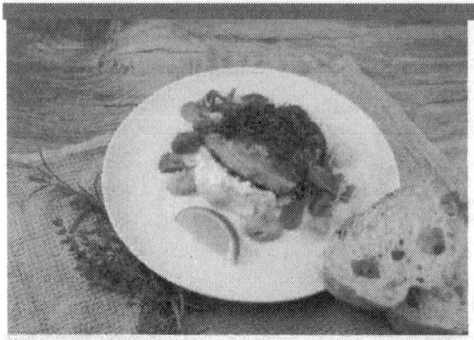

Preparation: 5 min | **Cooking:** 0 min | **Servings:** 4

Ingredients:
- 2 bunches watercress
- 1-pound smoked salmon, skinless, boneless, and flaked
- 2 teaspoons mustard
- ¼ cup lemon juice
- ½ cup Greek yogurt
- Salt and black pepper to taste
- 1 big cucumber, sliced
- 2 tablespoons chives, chopped

Directions:
1. In a salad bowl, combine the salmon with the watercress and the rest of the ingredients.
2. Toss and serve right away.

Nutrition: Calories: 244 | Fats: 16.7 g | Carbs: 22.5 g | Protein: 15.6 g

Salmon and Corn Salad

Ingredients:
- ½ cup pecans, chopped
- 2 cups baby arugula
- 1 cup corn
- ¼ pound smoked salmon, skinless, boneless, and cut into small chunks
- 2 tablespoons olive oil
- 2 tablespoons lemon juice
- Sea salt and black pepper to taste

Preparation: 5 min | **Cooking:** 0 min | **Servings:** 4

Directions:
1. In a salad bowl, combine the salmon with the corn and the rest of the ingredients.
2. Toss and serve right away.

Nutrition: Calories: 284 | Fats: 18.4 g | Carbs: 22.6 g | Protein: 17.4 g

Feta and Pesto Wrap

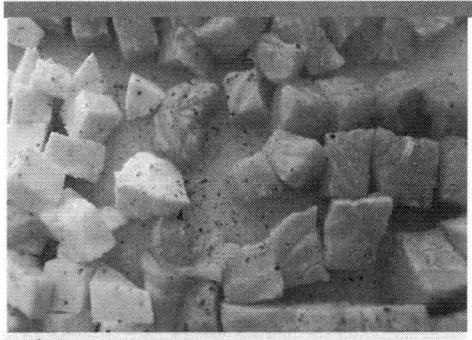

Preparation: 15 min
Cooking: 10 min
Servings: 4

Ingredients:
- 8 ounces (250 g) smoked salmon fillet, thinly sliced
- 1 cup (150 g) feta cheese
- 8 (15 g) Romaine lettuce leaves
- 4 (6-inch) pita bread
- ¼ cup (60 g) basil pesto sauce

Directions:
1. Place 1 pita bread on a plate.
2. Top with lettuce, salmon, feta cheese, and pesto sauce.
3. Fold or roll to enclose filling.
4. Repeat the procedure for the remaining ingredients.
5. Serve and enjoy.

Nutrition: Calories: 408 | Fats: 2g | Carbs: 1g | Protein: 11 g

Salmon Bowls

Preparation: 10 min
Cooking: 40 min
Servings: 3

Ingredients:
- 2 cups farro
- 2 lemons, juiced
- 1/3 cup olive oil + 2 tablespoons
- Salt and black pepper
- 1 cucumber, chopped
- ¼ cup balsamic vinegar
- 1 garlic clove, minced
- ¼ cup parsley, chopped
- ¼ cup mint, chopped
- 2 tablespoons mustard
- 4 salmon fillets, boneless

Directions:
1. In a large pot, boil water over medium-high heat. Add salt and the farro. Stir, simmer for 30 minutes, drain, and transfer to a bowl. Add the lemon juice, mustard, garlic, salt, pepper, and 1/3 cup oil. Toss and leave aside for now.
2. In another bowl, mash the cucumber with a fork. Add the vinegar, salt, pepper, parsley, dill, and mint; whisk well.
3. Heat a pan with the rest of the oil over medium fire. Add the salmon fillets, skin side down, and cook for 5 minutes on each side. Cool them down and break them into pieces.
4. Add over the farro; add the cucumber dressing, toss and serve for lunch.

Nutrition: Calories: 281 | Fats: 12.7g | Carbs: 5.8 g| Protein: 36.5g

Salmon with Vegetables

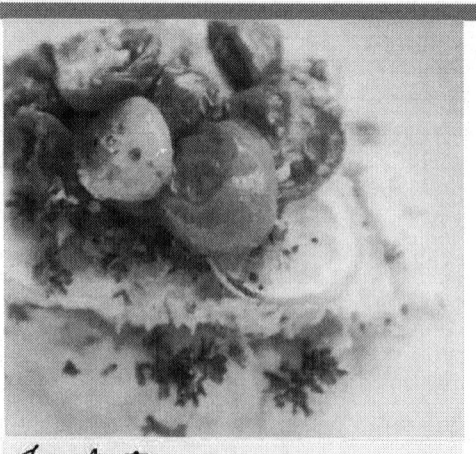

Preparation: 10 min
Cooking: 15 min
Servings: 4

Directions:

1. In a skillet, heat olive oil, and add fennel, squash, onion, ginger, and carrot. Cook until vegetables are soft.
2. Add wine, water, and parsley, and cook for another 4-5 minutes.
3. Season salmon fillets and place them in the pan.
4. Cook for 5 minutes per side or until it is ready.
5. Transfer salmon to a bowl, spoon tomatoes and scallion around salmon and serve.

Nutrition: Calories: 301 | Total Carbs: 2 g | Total Fats: 14 g | Protein: 13 g

Ingredients:

- 2 tablespoons olive oil
- 2 carrots
- 1 head fennel
- 2 squashes
- ¼ onion
- 1-inch ginger
- 1 cup white wine
- 2 cups water
- 2 parsley sprigs
- 2 tarragon sprigs
- 6 ounces salmon fillets
- 1 cup cherry tomatoes
- 1 scallion

Salmon Burgers

Ingredients:

- 1 lb. salmon fillets
- 1 onion
- ¼ dill fronds
- 1 tablespoon honey
- 1 tablespoon horseradish
- 1 tablespoon mustard
- 1 tablespoon olive oil
- 2 toasted split rolls
- 1 avocado

Preparation: 10 min
Cooking: 15 min
Servings: 4

Directions:

1. Place salmon fillets in a blender and blend until smooth. Transfer to a bowl, add onion, dill, honey, and horseradish, and mix well.
2. Add salt and pepper and form 4 patties.
3. In a bowl, combine mustard, honey, mayonnaise, and dill.
4. In a skillet, heat oil. Add salmon patties and cook for 2-3 minutes per side.
5. When ready, remove from heat.
6. Divide lettuce and onion between the buns.
7. Place salmon patty on top and spoon mustard mixture and avocado slices.
8. Serve when ready.

Nutrition: Calories: 189 | Total Carbs: 6 g | Total Fats: 7 g | Protein: 12 g

Black Cod

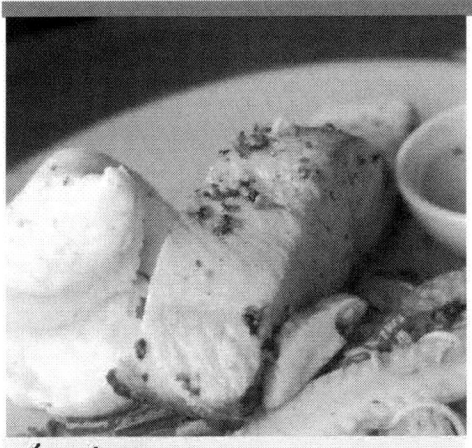

Preparation: 15 min | **Cooking:** 20 min | **Servings:** 4

Directions:

1. In a bowl, combine miso, soy sauce, and oil.
2. Rub the mixture over cod fillets and let it marinade for 20-30 minutes.
3. Adjust broiler and broil cod filets for 10-12 minutes.
4. When fish is cooked, remove and serve.

Nutrition: Calories: 281 | Total Carbs: 2 g | Total Fats: 10 g | Protein: 16 g

Ingredients:

- ¼ cup miso paste
- 1 tablespoon mirin
- 1 teaspoon soy sauce
- 1 tablespoon olive oil
- 4 black cod filets

Miso-Glazed Salmon

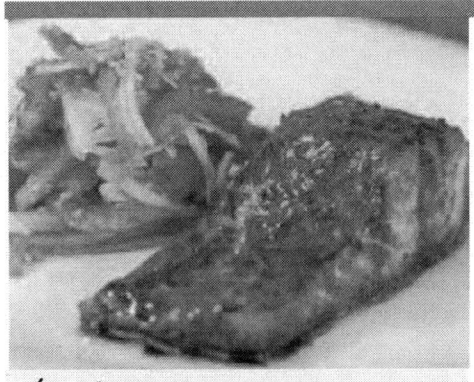

Preparation: 10 min | **Cooking:** 40 min | **Servings:** 4

Directions:

1. In a bowl, combine oil, soy sauce, and miso.
2. Rub the mixture over salmon fillets and marinade for 20-30 minutes.
3. Preheat a broiler.
4. Broil salmon for 5-10 minutes.
5. When ready, remove and serve.

Nutrition: Calories: 198 | Total Carbs: 5 g | Total Fats: 10 g | Protein: 6 g

Ingredients:

- ¼ cup red miso
- 1 tablespoon soy sauce
- 1 tablespoon vegetable oil
- 4 salmon fillets

Niçoise Salad

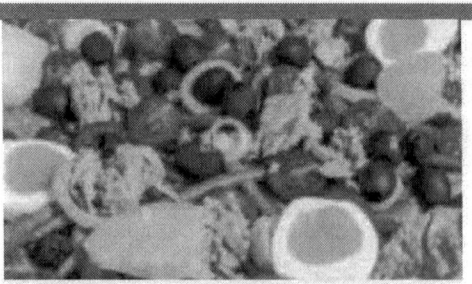

Preparation: 15 min
Cooking: 10 min
Servings: 4

Ingredients:
- 1-ounce red potatoes
- 1 package green beans
- 2 eggs
- ½ cup tomatoes
- 2 tablespoons wine vinegar
- ¼ teaspoon salt
- ½ teaspoon pepper
- ½ teaspoon thyme
- ¼ cup olive oil
- 6 ounces tuna
- ¼ cup Kalamata olives

Directions:
1. In a bowl, combine all ingredients.
2. Add salad dressing and serve.

Nutrition: Calories: 189 | Total Carbs: 2 g | Total Fats: 7 g | Protein: 15 g

Baked Fish With Feta and Tomato

Preparation: 5 min
Cooking: 15 min
Servings: 2

Ingredients:
- 2 pacific whitening fillets
- 1 scallion, chopped
- 1 Roma tomato, chopped
- 1 teaspoon fresh oregano
- 1-ounce feta cheese, crumbled

Seasoning:
- 2 tablespoons avocado oil
- 1/3 teaspoon salt
- ¼ teaspoon ground black pepper
- ¼ crushed red pepper

Directions:
1. Preheat the oven to 400°F.
2. Take a medium skillet pan, and place it over medium heat. Add oil and when hot, add scallion and cook for 3 minutes.
3. Add tomatoes, stir in ½ teaspoon of oregano, 1/8 teaspoon of salt, black pepper, and red pepper, pour in ¼ cup of water, and bring it to a simmer.
4. Sprinkle the remaining salt over the fillets. Add to the pan, drizzle with the remaining oil, and then bake for 10 to 12 minutes until fillets are fork-tender.
5. When done, top the fish with the remaining oregano and cheese and serve.

Nutrition: Calories: 427.5 | Fats: 29.5 g | Protein: 26.7 g | Net carb: 8 g

Salmon Panatela

Ingredients:

- 1 lb. skinned salmon, cut into 4 steaks each
- 1 cucumber, peeled, seeded, cubed
- Salt and black pepper to taste
- 8 black olives, pitted and chopped
- 1 tablespoon capers, rinsed
- 2 large tomatoes, diced
- 3 tablespoons red wine vinegar
- ¼ cup thinly sliced red onion
- 3 tablespoons olive oil
- 2 slices zero-carb bread, cubed
- ¼ cup thinly sliced basil leaves

Preparation: 5 min
Cooking: 22 min
Servings: 4

Directions:

1. Preheat a grill to 350°F and prepare the salad. In a bowl, mix the cucumbers, olives, pepper, capers, tomatoes, wine vinegar, onion, olive oil, bread, and basil leaves. Let it sit for the flavors to incorporate.
2. Season the salmon steaks with salt and pepper; grill them on both sides for 8 minutes. Serve the salmon steaks warm on a bed of veggies salad.

Nutrition: Calories: 338 | Fat: 27 g | Net Carbs: 1 g | Protein: 25 g

Shrimp Fried "Rice"

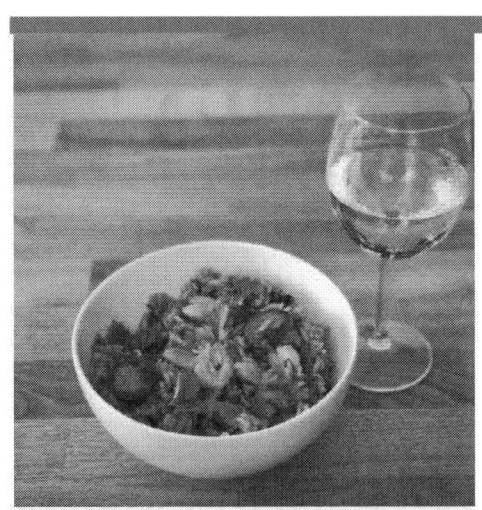

Preparation: 10 min
Cooking: 15 min
Servings: 4

Directions:

1. Heat 2 tablespoons of coconut oil in a large skillet over a high fire. Add shrimp and cook for 2-4 minutes until opaque and pink.
2. Remove from pan and set aside.
3. Add 2 tablespoons of coconut oil and add the cauliflower, peppers, and green onions.
4. Sautee for 4-5 minutes, stirring frequently.
5. Add the eggs and soy sauce to the pan and stir continuously until the eggs are firm.
6. Add the toasted sesame oil and stir; then toss with the shrimp and serve.

Nutrition: Calories: 482 | Carbs: 44.5 g | Protein: 29.5 g | Fat: 15 g

Ingredients:

- 2 + 2 tablespoons coconut oil
- 3 cups grated cauliflower
- 2 bell peppers, chopped
- 6 green onions, thinly sliced
- 1 lb. shrimp
- 4 eggs, lightly beaten
- 1 tablespoon soy sauce
- 2 tablespoons toasted sesame oil

Barbecued Spiced Tuna With Avocado-Mango Salsa

Ingredients:

- 4 (120 g each) skinless tuna fillets
- 1 teaspoon dried oregano
- 1 teaspoon onion powder
- 1 teaspoon ground paprika
- 1 teaspoon ground coriander
- 1 teaspoon ground cumin
- 1 tablespoon olive oil
- Thinly shaved fennel
- Baby rocket leaves

Avocado-Mango Salsa:
- ½ red onion, chopped
- 1 cucumber, chopped
- 1 avocado, diced
- 1 mango, diced
- 1 long red chili, chopped
- 2 tablespoons lime juice
- ½ cup chopped coriander

Preparation: 10 min
Cooking: 10 min
Servings: 4

Directions:

1. In a bowl, mix onion powder, paprika, coriander, cumin, and oil until well combined; add in tuna and turn until well coated; sprinkle with salt and pepper.
2. Preheat the BBQ grill to medium-high and grill the fish for about 3 minutes per side or until cooked to your liking. Wrap in foil and let it sit for at least 5 minutes.
3. In the meantime, in a bowl, mix avocado, mango, red onion, cucumber, chili, coriander, and fresh lime juice until well combined.
4. Divide fennel and rocket on serving plates and top each with the grilled tuna and mango-avocado salsa. Serve right away.

Nutrition: Calories: 300 | Total Fats: 17 g | Total Carbs: 34 g | Protein: 7 g

Salmon Foil-Pack

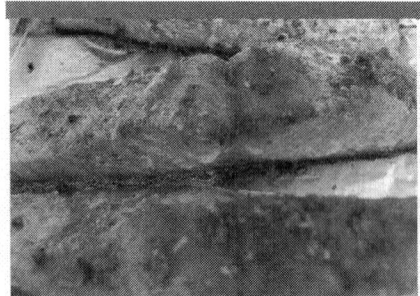

Ingredients:

- 1 salmon fillet
- 2 sheets nonstick aluminum foil
- 1 small yellow squash, cut into ¼-inch rounds
- 1 small sweet potato, peeled and sliced into ¼-inch slices
- 1 small zucchini, cut into ¼-inch rounds
- 1 ½ teaspoons smoky mesquite seasoning
- 1 lemon, cut into wedges

Preparation: 10 min
Cooking: 20 min
Servings: 1

Directions:

1. Preheat the oven to 400°F.
2. Prepare 2 large squares of foil, the nonstick side up, and let one be on top of the other.
3. Layer zucchini, potato, and squash in the center of the foil on the top, and then season each layer with mesquite season.
4. Place the salmon fillet on the layer, fold over the foil, and seal the packet tightly.
5. Place it in the oven and bake for 20 minutes or until the salmon fillet flakes easily with a fork.
6. Remove from oven and serve with lemon wedges.

Nutrition: Calories: 377 | Protein: 35.6 g | Carbs: 40.4 g | Fats: 9.1 g

Yummy Cedar Planked Salmon

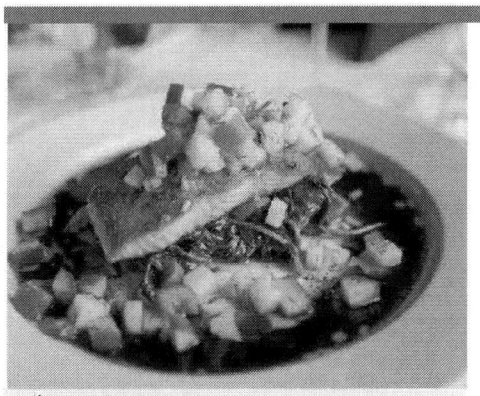

Preparation: 30 min
Cooking: 20 min
Servings: 6

Directions:

1. Pour warm water into a medium bowl, add the cedar planks, and let it soak for 1 hour or more, if possible.
2. Combine the olive oil, rice vinegar, green onions, ginger, garlic sesame oil, and soy sauce in a shallow dish and stir well.
3. Put the salmon fish in the mixture and turn well coated. Cover and let it marinate for 30 minutes to 1 hour.
4. Preheat the grill gas to medium fire and place the cedar planks on the grate. When the board starts to smoke and crackle, that shows it is ready.
5. Remove the salmon fish from the marinade and discard the marinade. Place the salmon fish onto the cedar planks and cover.
6. Place on a grill rack and bake for 20 minutes or until the fish flakes easily with a fork.
7. Remove from heat and serve with salad. Enjoy!

Nutrition: Calories: 678 | Protein: 61.3 g | Carbs: 1.7 g | Fats: 45.8 g

Ingredients:

- 2 salmon fillets, remove skin
- 3 untreated cedar planks (12")
- 1 teaspoon sesame oil
- 1/3 cup extra virgin olive oil
- 1 ½ tablespoons rice vinegar
- 1/3 cup soy sauce
- ¼ cup chopped green onions
- 1 tablespoon grated fresh ginger root
- 1 teaspoon minced garlic

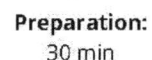

Quick Delicious Maple Salmon

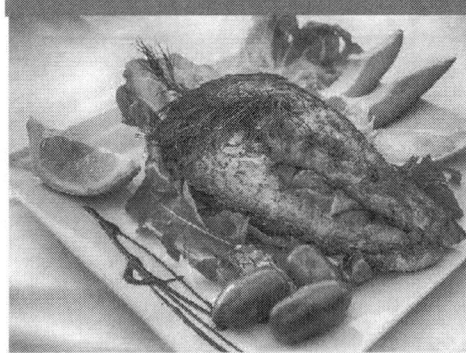

Preparation: 10 min
Cooking: 20 min
Servings: 4

Directions:

1. Preheat the oven to 400°F.
2. Combine the soy sauce, maple syrup, garlic, salt, and pepper and mix well.
3. Put the salmon fish in a glass baking dish. Add the soy sauce mixture and mix until well coated. Cover and put in the fridge for about 30 minutes.
4. Place the salmon in the heated oven and bake uncovered until it flakes easily with a fork, for about 20 minutes.
5. Remove from heat and serve.

Nutrition: Calories: 265 | Protein: 23.2 g | Carbs: 14.1 g | Fats: 45.8 g

Ingredients:

- 1 lb. salmon
- ¼ cup maple syrup
- 2 tablespoons soy sauce
- 1 garlic clove, minced
- ¼ teaspoons garlic salt
- 1/8 teaspoon freshly ground black pepper

Pan Seared Salmon

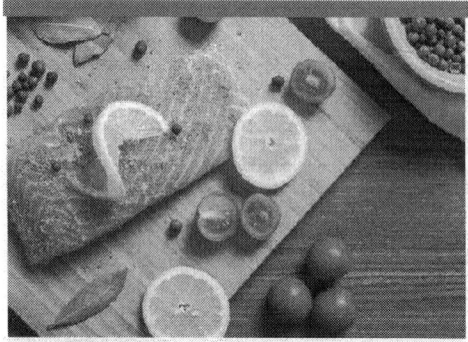

Preparation: 10 min

Cooking: 10 min

Servings: 4

Ingredients:

- 4 salmon fillets
- 2 tablespoons capers
- 2 tablespoons extra virgin olive oil
- 1/8 teaspoon salt
- 1/8 teaspoon freshly ground black pepper

Directions:

1. Preheat a large skillet over medium-high heat for about 3 minutes.
2. Properly coat the salmon fillets with oil and place them in the heated skillet.
3. Increase the heat to high heat and cook for 3 minutes. Sprinkle fish with caper, salt, and pepper.
4. Turn the salmon fish over and cook until the fish turns brown and flakes easily with a fork, for about 5 minutes more.
5. Divide among four serving plates and garnish with lemon slices.

Nutrition: Calories: 371 | Protein: 33.7 g | Carbs: 1.7 g | Fats: 25.1 g

Lemon Rosemary Salmon

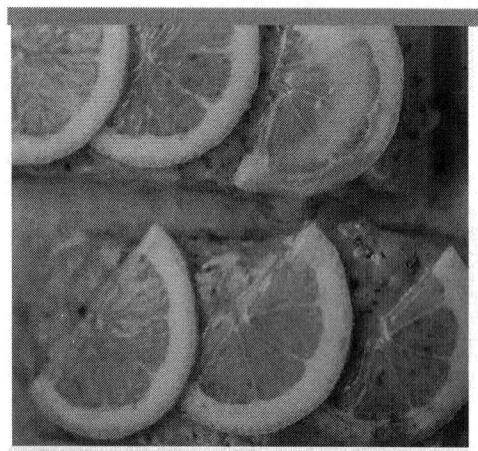

Preparation: 10 min

Cooking: 20 min

Servings: 4

Ingredients:

- 2 salmon fillets, bones, and skin removed
- 1 lemon, finely sliced
- 1 tablespoon extra-virgin olive oil
- 4 sprigs fresh rosemary
- Sea salt to taste

Directions:

1. Preheat the oven to 400°F.
2. On a baking sheet, arrange ½ of the lemon slices in a single layer.
3. Layer with the rosemary sprigs, place the fish on top, and sprinkle with salt, Layer with the rest of the lemon slices and drizzle with oil.
4. Place it in the oven and bake until the fish flakes easily with a fork, for about 20 minutes.
5. Remove from the oven and serve with crusty bread and salad.

Nutrition: Calories: 257 | Protein: 20.5 g | Carbs: 6.1 g | Fats: 18 g

Crispy Fish

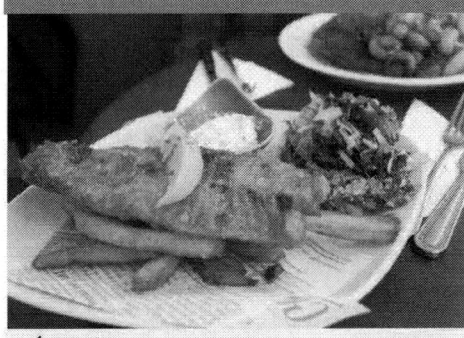

Preparation: 5 min
Cooking: 15 min
Servings: 4

Ingredients:
- Thick fish fillets
- ¼ cup all-purpose flour
- 1 egg
- 1 cup bread crumbs
- 2 tablespoons vegetables
- Lemon wedge

Directions:
1. Add flour, egg, and breadcrumbs to different dishes and set aside.
2. Dip each fish fillet into the flour, egg, and then bread crumbs bowl.
3. Place each fish fillet in a heated skillet and cook for 4-5 minutes per side.
4. When ready, remove from the pan and serve with lemon wedges.

Nutrition: Calories: 189 | Total Carbs: 2 | Total Fats: 17 g | Protein: 7 g

Tuna Noodle Casserole

Ingredients:
- 2 ounces egg noodles
- 4 ounces Fraiche
- 1 egg
- 1 teaspoon cornstarch
- 1 tablespoon juice from 1 lemon
- 1 can tuna
- 1 cup peas
- ¼ cup parsley

Preparation: 15 min
Cooking: 20 min
Servings: 4

Directions:
1. Boil the noodles in a saucepan with water.
2. In a bowl, combine egg, crème Fraiche and lemon juice, and whisk well.
3. When the noodles are cooked, add crème Fraiche mixture to the skillet and mix well.
4. Add tuna, peas, parsley, and lemon juice and mix well.
5. Bake for 10 minutes in the oven.
6. When ready, remove from heat and serve.

Nutrition: Calories: 214 | Total Carbs: 2 g | Total Fats: 7 g | Protein: 19 g

Seared Scallops

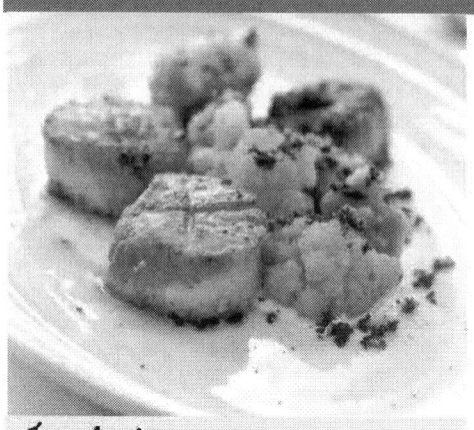

Preparation: 15 min
Cooking: 20 min
Servings: 4

Directions:

1. Season scallops and refrigerate for a couple of minutes.
2. In a skillet, heat oil, add scallops, and cook for 1-2 minutes per side.
3. When ready, remove from heat and serve.

Nutrition: Calories: 283 | Total Carbs: 10 g | Total Fats: 8 g | Protein: 9 g

Ingredients:

- 1 lb. sea scallops
- 1 tablespoon canola oil

Salmon Pasta

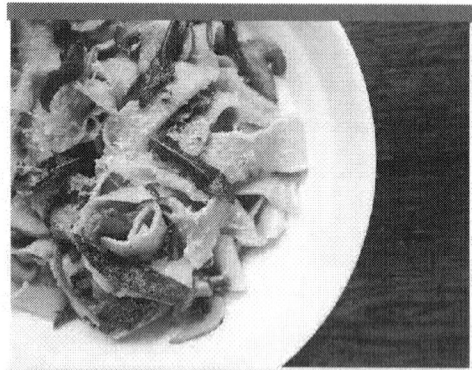

Preparation: 10 min
Cooking: 25 min
Servings: 2

Directions:

1. Bring a pot with water to a boil.
2. Add pasta and cook for 10-12 minutes.
3. In a skillet, add oil, and onion, and sauté until tender.
4. Stir in garlic powder, flour, milk, and cheese.
5. Add mushrooms and peas; cook on low heat for 4-5 minutes.
6. Toss in salmon and cook for another 2-3 minutes.
7. When ready, serve with cooked pasta.

Nutrition: Calories: 211 | Total Carbs: 7 g | Total Fats: 18 g | Protein: 17 g

Ingredients:

- 5 tablespoons olive oil
- ¼ onion
- 1 tablespoon all-purpose flour
- 1 teaspoon garlic powder
- 2 cups skim milk
- ¼ cup Romano cheese
- 1 cup green peas
- ¼ cup canned mushrooms
- 8 ounces salmon
- 1 package tagliatelle pasta

Crusty Pesto Salmon

Ingredients:
- ¼ cup roughly chopped pinoli
- ¼ cup pesto
- 2 x 4-ounces salmon fillets
- 2 tablespoons olive oil

Preparation: 5 min | **Cooking:** 15 min | **Servings:** 2

Directions:
1. Mix the pinoli and pesto together.
2. Place the salmon fillets in a round baking dish, roughly six inches in diameter.
3. Brush the fillets with oil, followed by the pesto mixture, ensuring to coat both the top and bottom. Put the baking dish inside the fryer.
4. Cook for twelve minutes at 390°F.
5. The salmon is ready when it flakes easily when prodded with a fork. Serve warm.

Nutrition: Calories: 290 | Fats: 11 g | Protein: 20 g

Sesame Tuna Steak

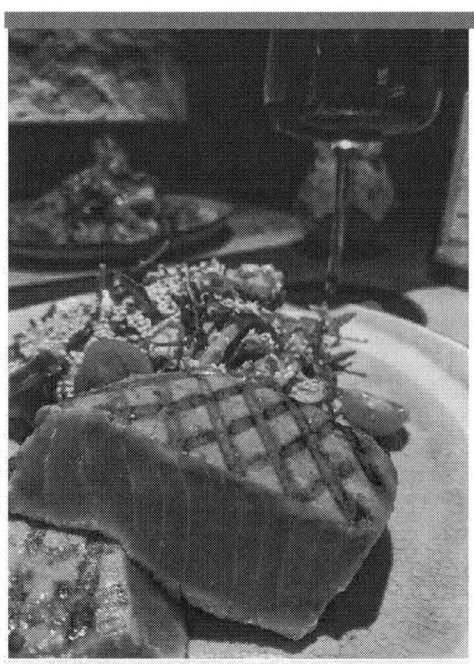

Preparation: 5 min | **Cooking:** 12 min | **Servings:** 2

Directions:
1. Apply the coconut oil to the tuna steaks; then season with garlic powder.
2. Combine the black and white sesame seeds.
3. Embed them in the tuna steaks, covering the fish all over.
4. Place the tuna into your Air Fryer.
5. Cook for eight minutes at 400°F, turning the fish halfway through.
6. The tuna steaks are ready when they have reached a temperature of 145°F.
7. Serve.

Nutrition: Calories: 160 | Fats: 6 g | Protein: 26 g

Ingredients:
- 1 tablespoon coconut oil, melted
- 2 x 6-ounces tuna steaks
- ½ teaspoon garlic powder
- 2 teaspoons black sesame seeds
- 2 teaspoons white sesame seeds

Foil Packet Lobster Tail

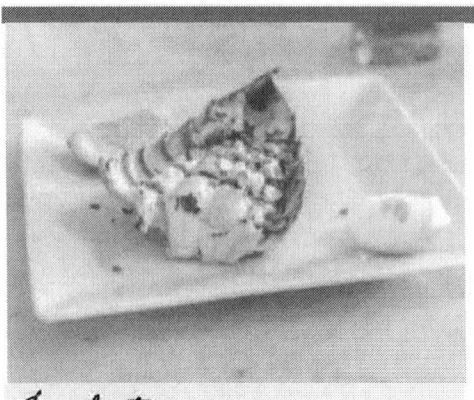

Preparation: 5 min

Cooking: 15 min

Servings: 2

Ingredients:

- 2 x 6-ounces lobster tail halves
- 2 tablespoons olive oil
- ½ medium lemon, juiced
- ½ teaspoon Old Bay seasoning
- 1 teaspoon dried parsley

Directions:

1. Lay each lobster on a sheet of aluminum foil. Pour a drizzle of olive oil and lemon juice over each one, and season with Old Bay.
2. Fold down the sides and ends of the foil to seal the lobster. Place each one in the fryer.
3. Cook at 375°F for twelve minutes.
4. Just before serving, top the lobster with dried parsley.

Nutrition: Calories: 510 | Fats: 18 g | Protein: 26 g

Soups & Stews

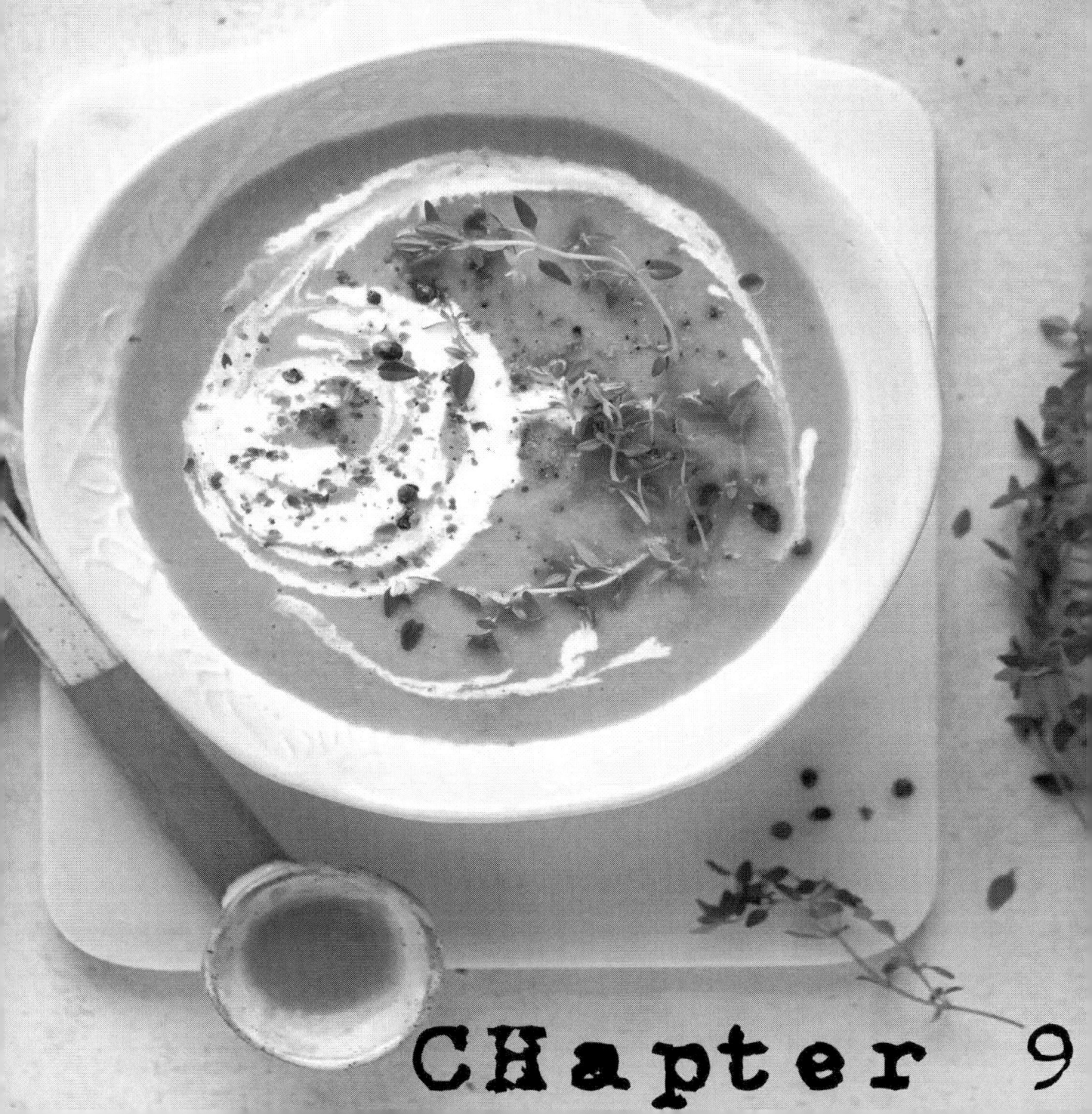

Chapter 9

Grilled Tomatoes Soup

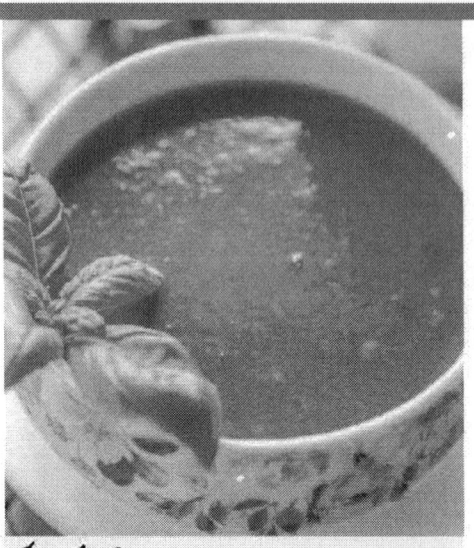

Preparation: 10 min | **Cooking:** 20 min | **Servings:** 1

Directions:
1. Cut the tomatoes into halves and grill them at 390°F for 1 minute from each side.
2. After this, transfer the grilled tomatoes to the blender and blend until smooth.
3. Place the shallot and avocado oil in the saucepan and roast it until light brown.
4. Add blended grilled tomatoes, ground black pepper, and minced garlic.
5. Bring the soup to a boil and sprinkle with dried basil.
6. Simmer the soup for 2 minutes more.

Nutrition: Calories: 72 | Protein: 4.1 g | Carbs: 13.4 g | Fats: 0.9 g

Ingredients:
- 2-pounds tomatoes
- ½ cup shallot, chopped
- 1 tablespoon avocado oil
- ½ teaspoon ground black pepper
- ¼ teaspoon minced garlic
- 1 tablespoon dried basil
- 3 cups low-sodium chicken broth

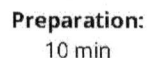

Lean Mean Soup

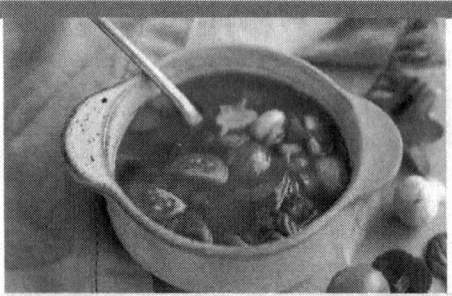

Preparation: 15 min | **Cooking:** 30 min | **Servings:** 6

Directions:
1. Add all the green soup ingredients to a cooking pot.
2. Cook for 30 minutes on low heat until veggies are soft.
3. Serve warm.

Serving Suggestion: Serve the soup with cauliflower rice.
Variation tip: Add broccoli florets to the soup as well.
Nutrition: Calories: 114 | Fats: 2.2 g | Carbs: 27.7 g | Protein: 8.8 g

Ingredients:
- ½ head cabbage, chopped
- 3 cups broccoli, chopped
- 1 cup carrots, diced
- 8 stalks celery, diced
- 1 cup onion, diced
- 1 cup radishes, chopped
- ½ cup yellow pepper, diced
- ½ cup red pepper, diced
- ½ cup orange pepper, diced
- 2 tablespoons garlic, minced
- 1 - 6 ounce can tomato paste
- 2 - 14-ounce cans diced tomatoes with green chiles, undrained
- 6 ½ cups water
- 1 teaspoon dried parsley
- 1 teaspoon dried oregano
- 1 teaspoon turmeric
- ½ cup kale
- Salt and black pepper to taste

Crockpot Lentil Soup

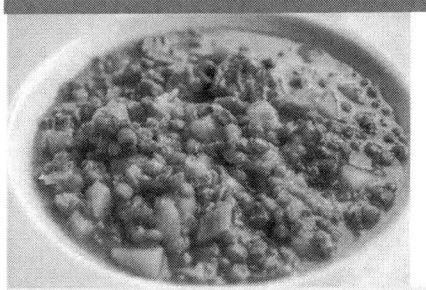

Preparation: 30 min
Cooking: 5 hrs 30 min
Servings: 8

Ingredients:

For the Crockpot:
- 2 cups butternut squash peeled and cubed
- 2 cups carrots peeled and sliced
- 1 cup green lentils
- 2 cups potatoes, finely chopped
- 2 cups celery, finely chopped
- ¾ cup yellow split peas
- 1 onion finely chopped
- 2 teaspoons herb de Provence
- 5 garlic cloves, minced
- 8 - 10 cups chicken broth
- 1 teaspoon salt
- 2-3 cups kale (removes steam and thinly chopped)
- 1 cup parsley (finely chopped)
- ½ cup olive oil
- 1 tablespoon lemon juice

Directions:

1. Combine all the ingredients in a Crockpot; close the lid and cook for 5 hours on high heat or 8 hours on low heat.
2. In a high-power blender, place 4 cups of the soup, add olive oil and blend until roughly smooth.
3. Return the soup to the pot and stir well. Add the parsley and kale; stir well.
4. Remove from heat and let it cool to room temperature.
5. Top with vinegar, sherry, and lemon juice; then serve with crusty wheat bread. Enjoy!

Nutrition: Calories: 322 | Protein: 10.8 g | Carbs: 39.5 g | Fats: 14 g

Turmeric Chicken Soup

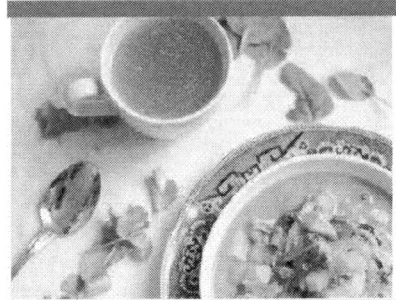

Preparation: 20 min
Cooking: 50 min
Servings: 12

Ingredients:

- 1 ½ pounds chicken breast, boneless and skinless
- 3 cups broccoli florets
- 2 quarts chicken broth
- ¼ cup chopped parsley
- 2 ½ cups sliced carrots
- ¼ teaspoon ground turmeric
- 1 large onion, finely chopped
- 2 tablespoons olive oil
- 2 cups chopped celery
- ¼ - ½ teaspoons crushed red pepper
- 1 ½ cups frozen peas
- 3 tablespoons fresh ginger, shredded or grated
- 4 garlic cloves minced
- 1 tablespoon apple cider vinegar
- Sea salt to taste
- Freshly ground pepper to taste

Directions:

1. Heat the oil in a saucepan over medium heat; add onions, ginger, celery, and garlic and cook until softened, for 6 minutes
2. Add the chicken, apple cider vinegar, carrots, turmeric, crushed red pepper, broth, and salt to taste.
3. Lower the heat to low and let it simmer until the chicken is cooked about 20-22 minutes.
4. Carefully remove the chicken with tongs to a chopping board to cool down.
5. Add the broccoli, parsley, and peas to the pot and let it simmer for 8 minutes until the broccoli is softened.
6. Shred or slice the chicken; return it to the pot soup and let it simmer for 12 minutes until the broccoli is softened, Season with salt and pepper to taste.
7. Scoop to a serving plate and serve immediately. Enjoy!

Nutrition: Calories: 91 | Protein: 9 g | Carbs: 65 g | Fats: 2 g

Healthy Silky Tortilla Soup

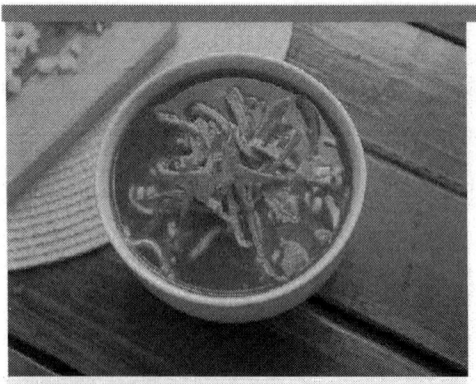

Preparation: 15 min
Cooking: 20 min
Servings: 5

Directions:

1. Heat 1 tablespoon of oil in a skillet, add onions, garlic, jalapeno, and red pepper to the skillet; cook for 4 minutes.
2. Transfer to a blender and add the vegetable broth, salsa, roasted black beans, and tomatoes. Pulse on speed until puree, for about six times.
3. Return to a pot and simmer on medium heat for 15 minutes.
4. In a heavy skillet, heat the 2 tablespoons of oil, add the tortilla chips, and fry until crisp. Drain chips on a paper towel until ready to use.
5. Divide soup among five serving plates and top with tortilla strips, shredded chicken, cheese, and fresh pepper. Enjoy!

Nutrition: Calories: 350 | Protein: 13 g | Carbs: 25 g | Fats: 14 g

Ingredients:

- 3 tablespoons extra virgin olive oil, divided
- 3 cloves garlic
- 1 cup white onion, finely chopped
- 1 jalapeno pepper Remove seed and finely chopped
- ½ teaspoon red pepper flakes
- 12 ounces salsa
- 1 ½ cups vegetable broth
- 14.5 ounces fire-roasted tomatoes
- ½ cup black beans
- 1 lb. chicken breast, cooked and shredded
- Jalapeno peppers, sliced fresh
- 3 corn tortillas cut into thin strips
- Shredded cheddar cheese

Healthy Carrot Ginger Soup

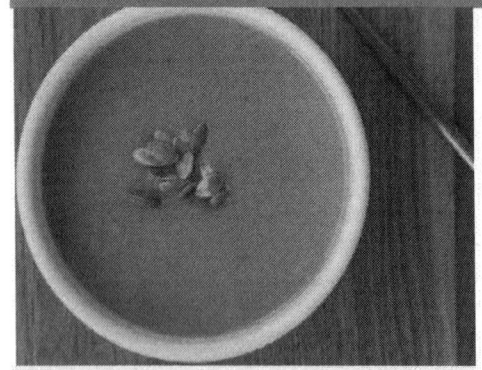

Preparation: 20 min
Cooking: 40 min
Servings: 4

Directions:

1. Heat oil in a large saucepan over medium-high fire. Add onion, garlic, and ¼ teaspoon of salt; cook until onion is softened and translucent, for about 5 minutes.
2. Add ginger and carrot to the saucepan and cook until equally coated and fragrant for 1 minute.
3. Add the broth and the rest of the salt and let it boil over high heat
4. Lower the heat to medium. Partially cover the saucepan and let it simmer until the carrot is softened, for about 20 minutes.
5. Remove from heat and add ½ cup of almond milk and let it slightly cool down.
6. Transfer to a blender and blend on high until smooth and creamy, for about 1 minute (you can blend in batches).
7. Return to the saucepan, taste, and adjust season; then warm on low heat.
8. Spoon soup on a serving plate, add the remaining almond milk, and swirl it with a butter knife. Enjoy!

Nutrition: Calories: 220 | Protein: 10 g | Carbs: 27 g | Fats: 16 g

Ingredients:

- 6 cups carrots, peeled and cubed
- 2 tablespoons extra-virgin olive oil
- 2 cups diced yellow onion
- 5 cups vegetable broth
- 2 teaspoons minced garlic
- 2 tablespoons minced fresh ginger
- ¾ cup full-fat canned almond milk
- 1 teaspoon sea salt

Chicken Tortilla Avocado Soup

Ingredients:

- 2 garlic cloves, finely chopped
- 1 tablespoon extra-virgin olive oil
- 1 corn tortilla, 7" in length, torn into pieces
- 1 medium yellow onion, finely chopped
- 15 ounces diced fire-roasted tomatoes with juice
- 4 oz. diced mild green chilies
- 2 cups chicken stock
- 2 teaspoons chili powder
- 1 teaspoon ground cumin
- 1 lime (juiced and peel grated)
- ¼ cup chopped fresh cilantro
- 1 cup tortilla chips
- 2 cups cooked chicken, chopped
- 1 avocado, halved, pitted, peeled, and diced
- Sea salt to taste

Preparation: 10 min
Cooking: 10 min
Servings: 5

Directions:

1. Heat the olive oil in a skillet over a medium-high fire and add onion, garlic, and a little salt. Cover the skillet and cook until softened, for about 8 minutes. Remove from heat and set aside to cool.
2. Combine the torn tortilla, chiles, tomatoes, stock, cumin, chili powder, lime peel, cilantro, juice, and 1 teaspoon of salt in the blender bowl. Add the onion and garlic mixture to the blender and cover with a lid.
3. Start from the lowest speed and slowly increase to the highest. Blend for 5 minutes or until the mixture is smooth and rising steam is noticeable.
4. Add the tortilla chips and chicken to the blender bowl and pulse 3 times.
5. Spoon onto a serving plate, garnish with cheese and avocado slices; then serve immediately. Enjoy!
6. Note: to store, let the tortilla chips cool off completely, then transfer them to an airtight container and store them in the fridge. Make sure you consume it within a week. You can also freeze for up to 3 months. Add tortilla chips when warming.

Nutrition: Calories: 370 | Protein: 24 g | Carbs: 27 g | Fats: 22 g |

Spicy Chicken and Kale

Ingredients:

- 2 tablespoons extra virgin olive oil
- 1 red onion (peeled and chopped)
- 1 fennel bulb (cored and sliced)
- 3 cloves garlic (minced)
- 1 ½ lb. chicken breast, cut into bite-size pieces
- 3 ½ cups diced tomatoes
- 4 cups chicken broth
- 1 cup dry white wine
- 4 cups kale (chopped)
- ¼ teaspoon crushed red pepper
- 6 ounces plain Greek yogurt
- 1 ½ tablespoon extra virgin olive oil
- 1 cup basil leaves
- Sea salt to taste
- Freshly ground black pepper

Preparation: 15 min
Cooking: 30 min
Servings: 5

Directions:

1. Heat oil in a large pot over a medium-high fire. Add onions and fennel to the pot and cook for 4 minutes. Add garlic and cook until the veggies are softened, for about more 3 minutes
2. Remove the veggies or push them aside; add the chicken and heat until almost cooked, for 5 minutes.
3. Add the chicken broth, tomatoes, kale, wine, red pepper, salt, and pepper to taste. Bring to boil over medium-high heat; reduce heat to medium-low and let it simmer for 20 minutes.
4. While the soup is simmering, Combine the oil, yogurt, and basil in a blender bowl. Add a pinch of salt and blend until smooth.
5. To serve, spoon soup on a serving plate with yogurt and basil mixture on top and enjoy!

Nutrition: Calories: 400 | Protein: 37 g | Carbs: 22 g | Fats: 17 g

Halibut Tomato Soup

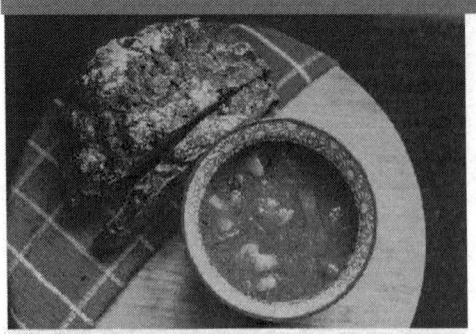

Preparation: 5 min
Cooking: 60 min
Servings: 2

Ingredients:

- 2 garlic cloves, minced
- 1 tablespoon olive oil
- ¼ cup fresh parsley, chopped
- 10 anchovies canned in oil, minced
- 6 cups vegetable broth
- 1 teaspoon black pepper
- 1 pound halibut fillets, chopped
- 3 tomatoes, peeled and diced
- 1 teaspoon salt
- 1 teaspoon red chili flakes

Directions:

1. Heat olive oil in a large stockpot over medium fire and add garlic and half of the parsley.
2. Add anchovies, tomatoes, vegetable broth, red chili flakes, salt, and black pepper, and bring to a boil.
3. Reduce the heat to medium-low and simmer for about 20 minutes.
4. Add halibut fillets and cook for about 10 minutes.
5. Dish out the halibut and shred it into small pieces.
6. Mix back with the soup and garnish with the remaining fresh parsley to serve.

Nutrition: Calories: 170 | Carbs: 3 g | Fats: 6.7 g | Protein: 23.4 g

Detox-Liver Arugula and Broccoli Soup

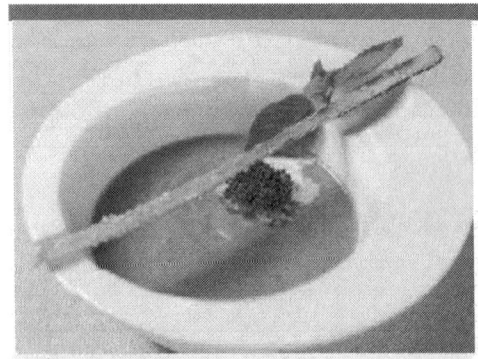

Preparation: 3 min
Cooking: 20 min
Servings: 4

Ingredients:

- 5 cups water
- 2 cups arugula leaves, packed
- ½ teaspoon thyme
- ½ teaspoon freshly ground black pepper
- 2 tablespoon olive oil
- ½ teaspoon salt
- 1 lemon juice
- 1 yellow or Spanish onion, roughly diced
- 2 garlic cloves, chopped
- 2 (about 4/6 pounds) head broccoli, cut into little florets

Directions:

1. Heat 2 tablespoons of olive oil over a medium flame in a large saucepan. Cook onion in the heated oil until soft and translucent.
2. Pour in chopped garlic and cook for 60 seconds, add broccoli and cook for about 4 minutes more or until it is bright green. Add ½ teaspoon of freshly ground black pepper, salt, thyme, and cups of water. Allow the mixture to heat through; lower the heat and cook with the lid on for about 8 minutes or until broccoli is tender.
3. Blend the soup in a blender or use an immersion blender. Add the arugula and blend until smooth. Serve with lemon juice.

Nutrition: Calories: 352 | Fats: 22.5 g | Carbs: 7.6 g | Protein: 10.4 g

Unique Lentil With Kale Soup

Ingredients:
- ½ cup wild rice
- ½ cup steel-cut oats or barley
- ½ cup lentils (any will do)
- 4 cups kale, chopped
- ½ cup French lentils
- 8 cups vegetarian broth

Preparation: 10 min
Cooking: 1 hrs 10 min
Servings: 2

Directions:
1. Cook the vegetarian broth in a soup pot over medium fire until heated. Add the other ingredients, and stir.
2. Simmer on low with the lid on for 45 minutes to 1 hour.
3. Add chopped kale, stir and simmer for 10 more minutes. Serve and enjoy.

Nutrition: Calories: 317 | Fats: 12.5 g | Carbs: 17.6 g | Protein: 17.4 g

Pasta Veggies Minestrone Soup

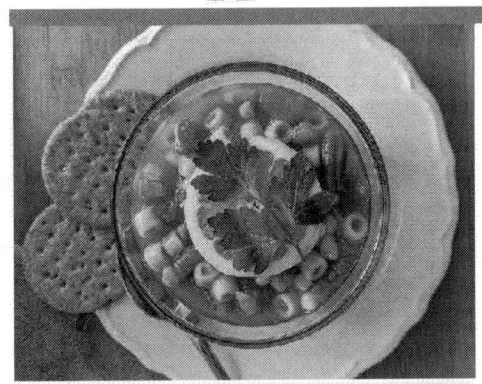

Preparation: 15 min
Cooking: 40 min
Servings: 2-4

Directions:
1. Heat a saucepan over medium fire.
2. Drizzle the saucepan with olive oil and sauté the chopped onion for about 4 minutes, stirring periodically until browned a bit. Except for the pasta, add in the rest ingredients and bring to a boil.
3. Reduce to low heat and simmer with the lid on for 25 minutes, stirring occasionally.
4. Add and cook pasta according to package instructions, about 10-12 minutes until pasta is al dente.

Nutrition: Calories: 352 | Fats: 12.5 g | Carbs: 7.6 g | Protein: 10.4 g

Ingredients:
- 1 tablespoon basil, finely chopped or 1 teaspoon dried basil
- 1 minced garlic clove
- 14-ounce can diced plum tomatoes
- 1/8 teaspoons salt
- 1/8 cup of your preferred pasta
- 1/16 teaspoon black pepper, freshly ground
- 3/8 cup diced celery
- ½ cup cannellini beans
- 1.5 cups water
- ½ cup carrots, peeled and sliced
- 1 cup diced zucchini
- 3/8 cup chopped onion
- ½ tablespoon extra-virgin olive oil
- 1/8 teaspoon dried oregano

Zucchini Noodles Soup

Ingredients:
- 2 zucchinis, trimmed
- 4 cups low-sodium chicken stock
- 2 ounces fresh parsley, chopped
- ½ teaspoon chili flakes
- 1 oz carrot, shredded
- 1 teaspoon olive oil

Preparation:	Cooking:	Servings:
10 min	15 min	2

Directions:

1. Roast the carrot with olive oil in the saucepan for 5 minutes over medium-low heat.
2. Stir it well and add chicken stock. Bring the mixture to a boil.
3. Meanwhile, make the noodles from the zucchini with the help of the spiralizer.
4. Add them to the boiling soup liquid.
5. Add parsley and chili flakes. Bring the soup to a boil and remove it from the heat.
6. Leave for 10 minutes to rest.

Nutrition: Calories 39 | Protein: 2.7 g | Carbs: 4.9 g | Fat: 1.5 g |

Chicken Oatmeal Soup

Ingredients:
- 1 cup oats
- 4 cups water
- 1-ounce fresh dill, chopped
- 10 ounces chicken fillet, chopped
- 1 teaspoon ground black pepper
- 1 teaspoon potato starch
- ½ carrot, diced

Preparation:	Cooking:	Servings:
10 min	15 min	2

Directions:

1. Put the chopped chicken in the saucepan, add water and bring it to a boil. Simmer the chicken for 10 minutes.
2. Add dill, ground black pepper, oats, and diced carrot.
3. Bring the soup to a boil and add potato starch. Stir it until the soup starts to thicken. Simmer the soup for 5 minutes on low heat.

Nutrition: Calories: 192 | Protein: 19.8 g | Carbs: 16.1 g | Fat: 5.5 g

Celery Cream Soup

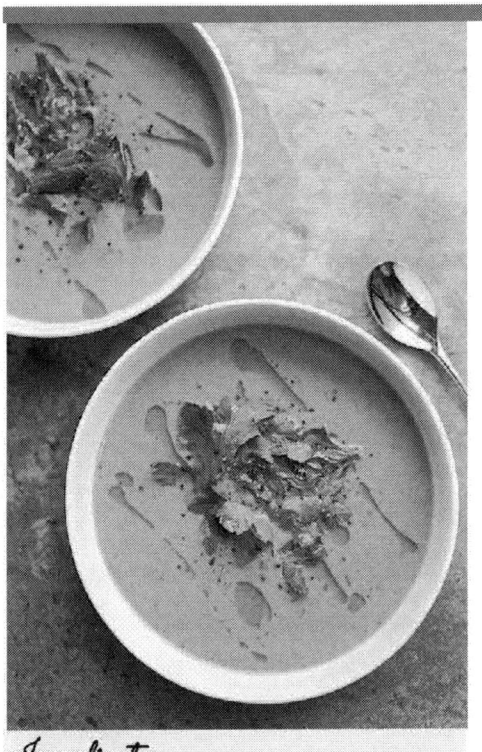

Preparation: 10 min | **Cooking:** 25 min | **Servings:** 1

Directions:

1. Melt the olive oil in the saucepan and add shallot and celery stalk. Cook the vegetables for 5 minutes. Stir them occasionally.
2. After this, add vegetable stock and potato.
3. Simmer the soup for 15 minutes.
4. Blend the soup tilly, get the creamy texture, and sprinkle with white pepper.
5. Simmer it for 5 minutes more.

Nutrition: Calories: 88 | Protein: 2.3 g | Carbs: 13.3 g | Fat: 3 g

Ingredients:

- 2 cups celery stalk, chopped
- 1 shallot, chopped
- 1 potato, chopped
- 4 cups low-sodium vegetable stock
- 1 tablespoon olive oil
- 1 teaspoon white pepper

Mint Quinoa

Ingredients:

- 1 cup quinoa
- 1 ¼ cup water
- 4 teaspoons lemon juice
- ¼ teaspoon garlic clove, diced
- 5 tablespoons sesame oil
- 2 cucumbers, chopped
- 1/3 teaspoon ground black pepper
- 1/3 cup tomatoes, chopped
- ½ ounce scallions, chopped
- ¼ teaspoon fresh mint, chopped

Preparation: 5 min | **Cooking:** 10 min | **Servings:** 2

Directions:

1. Pour water into the pan. Add quinoa and boil it for 10 minutes.
2. Then close the lid and let it rest for 5 minutes more.
3. Meanwhile, in the mixing bowl, mix up lemon juice, diced garlic, sesame oil, cucumbers, ground black pepper, tomatoes, scallions, and fresh mint.
4. Then add the cooked quinoa and carefully mix the side dish with the help of the spoon.
5. Store tabbouleh for up to 2 days in the fridge.

Nutrition: Calories: 168 | Fats: 9.9 | Carbs: 16.9 | Protein: 3.6

Pear Red Pepper Soup

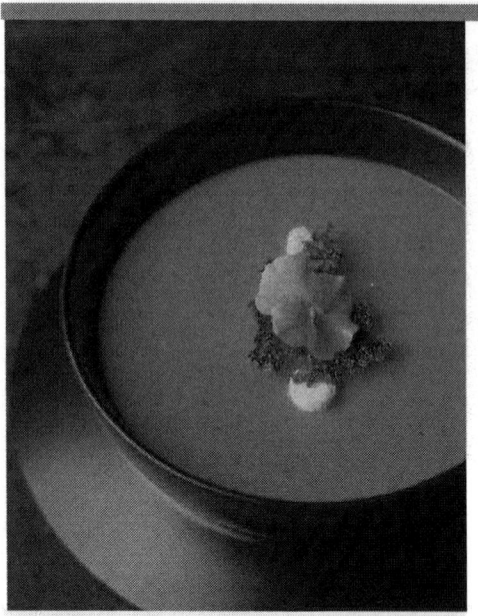

Preparation: 10 min
Cooking: 40 min
Servings: 4-5

Directions:

1. Heat the olive oil over medium heat in a Dutch oven; add bell pepper, carrots, shallots, and Anjou pears and sauté until tender, about 8 to 10 minutes.
2. Stir in chicken broth and all the peppers, and add salt. Cook until heated through. Cover with a lid and simmer on low heat for 25 to 30 minutes. Allow cooling for 20 minutes.
3. In the bowl of a food processor, add and process soup in batches until smooth, scraping the sides down as necessary. Transfer back to Dutch oven to keep warm until you are ready to use. Garnish, if desired.

Nutrition: Calories: 352 | Fats: 12.5 g | Carbs: 7.6 g | Protein: 10.4 g

Ingredients:

- 1 sliced shallot
- ¼ teaspoon of dried crushed red pepper
- 1 (16-ounce) container of no-fat chicken broth
- ¼ teaspoon of ground black pepper
- A pinch ground red pepper
- 1 peeled and sliced Anjou pear
- 1 ½ large sliced red bell peppers
- 1 teaspoon of olive oil
- 1/8 teaspoon of salt
- Garnishes (optional): fresh thinly sliced pears, chopped fresh chives, plain yogurt
- 1 sliced carrot

Low Heat Chicken Provençal

Ingredients:

- ¼ teaspoons freshly ground black pepper
- 2 (16-ounces each) can cannellini beans, rinsed and drained
- 2 teaspoons dried thyme
- 2 diced red pepper
- 2 diced yellow pepper
- 2 (14.5-ounce each) can petite diced tomatoes with basil, oregano, and garlic, undrained
- ¼ teaspoon salt
- 4 teaspoons dried basil
- 12 ounces (skins removed) bone-in chicken breast halves

Preparation: 5 min
Cooking: 8 hrs
Servings: 8

Directions:

1. Arrange the chicken in a crock pot; add the rest ingredients into the pot.
2. Cook with the lid on for 8 hours in a low-heat setting.

Nutrition: Calories: 85 | Fats: 6.5 g | Carbs: 0.6 g | Protein: 6.4 g

Danny's Tortellini Soup

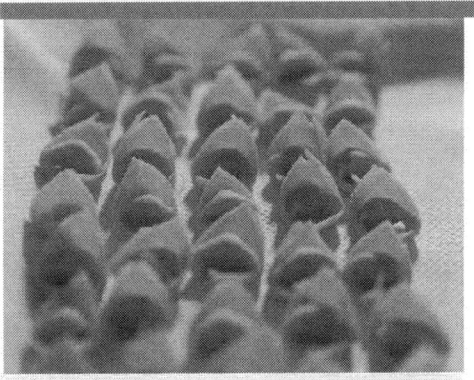

Preparation: 8 min | **Cooking:** 25 min | **Servings:** 3

Directions:

1. Heat 1 tablespoon of olive oil over a medium fire in a large saucepan. Add in the scallions, diced potato, diced celery, carrots, and diced zucchini.
2. Sauté the vegetables for 10 minutes over medium heat, stirring frequently until the vegetables start to soften. Add the tomatoes, chicken stock, and salt. Increase the flame and bring it to a low boil.
3. Add the tortellini and cook for about 2 minutes (6 minutes if frozen), then simmer on low heat for 5 to 6 minutes more. Stir in the pepper.

Nutrition: Calories: 85 | Fats: 6.5 g | Carbs: 0.6 g | Protein: 6.4 g

Ingredients:

- ½ peeled and diced potato
- 6 oz fresh or frozen tortellini (meat or cheese filled)
- 1-quart low-sodium chicken stock
- 2 scallions
- ½ large can crushed tomatoes (Spice the tomatoes with oregano and basil)
- 1 tablespoon olive oil
- 1 medium carrot, peeled and diced
- 1 small diced zucchini
- Black pepper to taste
- ¼ teaspoon salt
- 1 diced celery stalk

Wellness Parsnip Soup

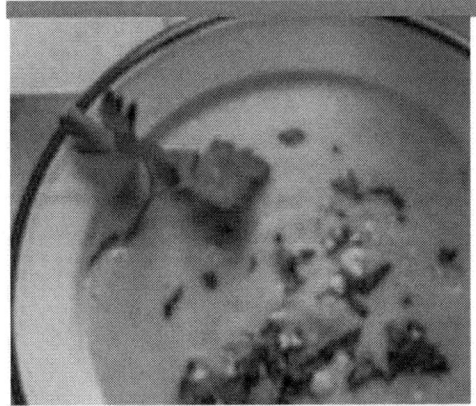

Preparation: 10 min | **Cooking:** 20 min | **Servings:** 6

Directions:

1. Heat 1 ½ tablespoon of olive oil over a medium flame in a large skillet. Sauté the onion and garlic in the pan for about 5 minutes until softened. Mix in the remaining ingredients, reserving only the broth or stock.
2. Cook and stir now and then for 2 minutes. Add stock or broth and cook until soup is heated through. Simmer on low heat until the vegetables are tender. Puree the soup with an immersion blender, serve and enjoy.

Nutrition: Calories: 85 | Fats: 6.5 g | Carbs: 0.6 g | Protein: 6.4 g

Ingredients:

- ¾ cup chopped pumpkin
- Salt and pepper to taste
- 1 ½ teaspoon ground cumin
- 7 ½ cups stock or broth
- 6 chopped medium parsnips
- 1 ½ tablespoons dried oregano
- 1 ½ tablespoon olive oil
- 4 ½ crushed garlic cloves
- 1 ½ finely chopped brown onion
- 3 chopped medium carrots

Feel Good Chicken Soup

Ingredients:
- 3 large diced carrots
- 3 bay leaves
- 1 ½ medium diced swede or turnip
- 3 sliced stalks celery
- 3 teaspoons dried oregano
- 1 ½ large sliced zucchini
- 3 tablespoons olive oil
- 7 ½ cups bone stock or broth
- 6 cups leftover cooked chicken, shredded
- 1 ½ cup canned coconut cream
- Salt and pepper
- 1 ½ small diced brown onion

Preparation: 10 min
Cooking: 10-15 min
Servings: 6

Directions:
1. Add 3 tablespoons of olive oil to a large pot, and sauté the vegetables until they are soft to your liking.
2. Add the remaining ingredients into the pot, reserving the coconut cream. When the vegetables are tender as desired, add coconut cream and stir to combine.
3. Turn the heat off and garnish with parsley.

Nutrition: Calories: 85 | Fats: 6.5 g | Carbs: 0.6 g | Protein: 6.4 g

Pork Soup

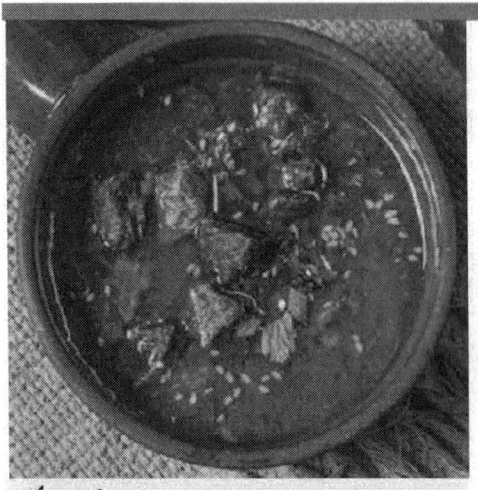

Preparation: 10 min
Cooking: 25 min
Servings: 2

Directions:
1. Heat a pot with the oil over a medium-high fire. Add the onion and pork, and cook the ingredients for 5 minutes.
2. Add all remaining ingredients and cook the soup for 20 minutes.

Nutrition: Calories: 304 | Protein: 34.5 g | Carbs: 14.2 g | Fats: 11.4 g

Ingredients:
- 1 tablespoon avocado oil
- 1 onion, chopped
- 1 pound pork stew meat, cubed
- 4 cups water
- 1-pound carrots, sliced
- 2 teaspoon tomato paste

Curry Soup

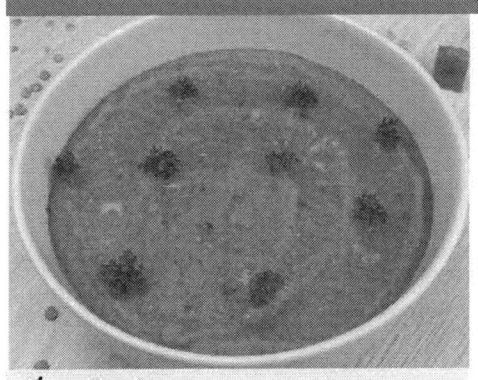

Preparation: 10 min
Cooking: 23 min
Servings: 2

Ingredients:
- 3 tablespoons olive oil
- 8 carrots, peeled and sliced
- 2 teaspoons curry paste
- 4 celery stalks, chopped
- 1 yellow onion, chopped
- 4 cups water

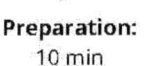

Directions:
1. Heat a pot with the oil and add onion, celery and carrots, stir and cook for 12 minutes.
2. Then add curry paste and water. Stir the soup well and cook it for 10 minutes more.
3. When all ingredients are soft, blend the soup until smooth and simmer it for 1 minute more.

Nutrition: Calories: 171 | Protein: 1.6 g | Carbs: 15.8 g | Fats: 12 g

Yellow Onion Soup

Preparation: 10 min
Cooking: 20 min
Servings: 2

Ingredients:
- 1 tablespoon avocado oil
- 1 yellow onion, chopped
- 1 teaspoon ginger, grated
- 1-pound zucchinis, chopped
- 4 cups low-sodium chicken broth
- ½ cup low-fat cream
- 1 teaspoon ground black pepper

Directions:
1. Heat a pot with the oil over medium fire. Add the onion and ginger, stir and cook for 5 minutes.
2. Add all remaining ingredients and simmer them over medium heat for 15 minutes.
3. Blend the cooked soup and ladle in the bowls.

Nutrition: Calories: 61 | Protein: 4.2 g | Carbs: 10.2 g | Fats: 0.7 g

Garlic Soup

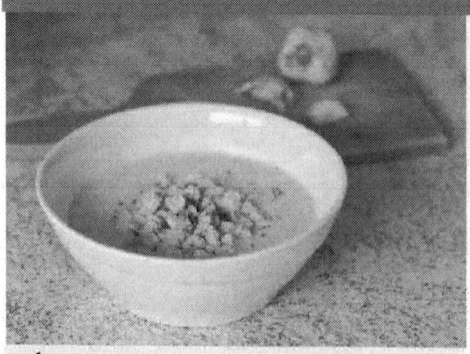

Preparation: 10 min

Cooking: 50 min

Servings: 2

Directions:

1. Pour water into a pot and heat up over medium heat.
2. Add all ingredients and close the lid.
3. Simmer the soup for 45 minutes over medium heat.

Nutrition: Calories: 620 | Protein: 60.9 g | Carbs: 75.8 g | Fats: 8.4 g

Ingredients:

- 1-pound red kidney beans, cooked
- 8 cups water
- 1 green bell pepper, chopped
- 1 tomato paste
- 1 yellow onion, chopped
- 1 teaspoon minced garlic
- 1 pound beef sirloin, cubed
- 1 teaspoon garlic powder

Chapter 10

Salads

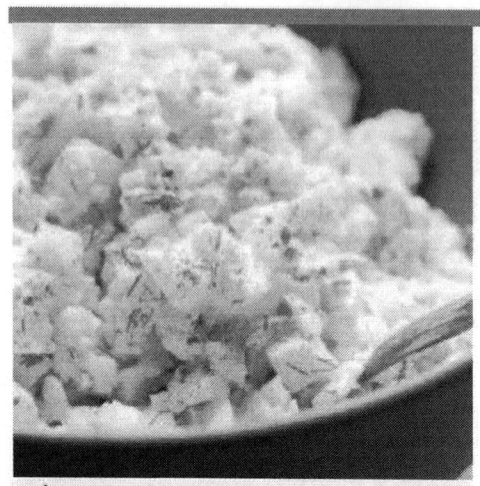

Cauliflower Salad

Preparation: 5 min
Cooking: 0 min
Servings: 4

Directions:

1. Toss cauliflower with seasoning and apple cider vinegar in a bowl.
2. Serve.

> Serving Suggestion: Serve the cauliflower salad with lemon wedges.
> Variation tip: Add chopped mushrooms and bell pepper to the salad as well.
> Nutrition: Calories: 93 | Fats: 3 g | Carbs: 12 g | Protein: 4 g

Ingredients:

- 4 cups cauliflower florets
- 1 tablespoon Tuscan fantasy seasoning
- ¼ cup apple cider vinegar

Avocado Tomato Salad

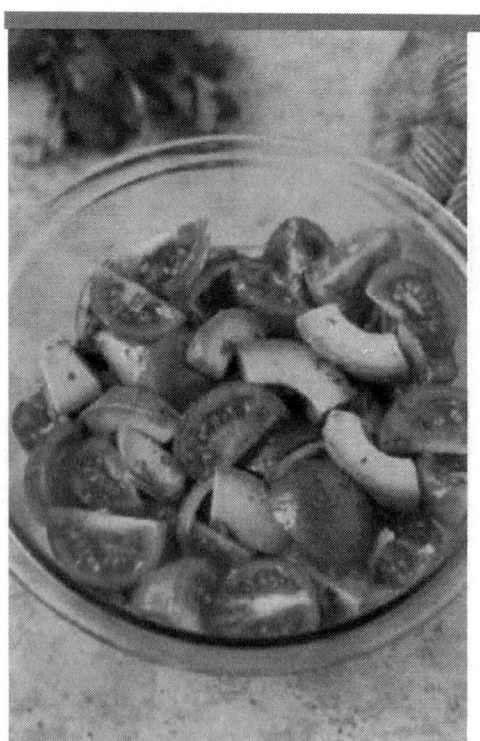

Preparation: 15 min
Cooking: 14 min
Servings: 2

Directions:

1. Peel the avocados, remove their pits, and cut them into cubes.
2. Transfer the avocados to a salad bowl.
3. Stir in tomatoes, lemon juice, cilantro, black pepper, and salt.
4. Mix well and serve fresh.

> Serving Suggestion: Serve the salad with grilled salmon.
> Variation tip: Add canned corn to the salad.
> Nutrition: Calories: 151 | Fats: 9 g | Carbs: 43 g | Protein: 3 g

Ingredients:

- 2 ripe avocados
- 2 ripe beefsteak tomatoes
- 2 tablespoons lemon juice
- 3 tablespoons cilantro, chopped
- Salt and black pepper to taste

Crispy Fennel Salad

Ingredients:
- 1 fennel bulb, finely sliced
- 1 grapefruit, cut into segments
- 1 orange, cut into segments
- 2 tablespoons almond slices, toasted
- 1 teaspoon chopped mint
- 1 tablespoon chopped dill
- Salt and pepper to taste
- 1 tablespoon grape seed oil

Preparation: 5 min | **Cooking:** 15 min | **Servings:** 2

Directions:
1. Mix the fennel bulb with the grapefruit and orange segments on a platter.
2. Top with almond slices, mint, and dill. Drizzle with the oil, and season with salt and pepper.
3. Serve the salad as fresh as possible.

Nutrition: Calories: 104 | Fats: 0.5 g | Protein: 3.1 g | Carbs: 25.5 g

Arugula and Sweet Potato Salad

Ingredients:
- 1 lb. sweet potatoes
- 1 cup walnuts
- 1 tablespoon olive oil
- 1 cup water
- 1 tablespoon soy sauce
- 3 cups arugula

Preparation: 10 min | **Cooking:** 20 min | **Servings:** 4

Directions:
1. Bake potatoes at 400°F until tender; remove and set aside.
2. In a bowl, drizzle walnuts with olive oil and microwave for 2-3 minutes or until toasted.
3. In a bowl, combine all salad ingredients and mix well.
4. Pour over the soy sauce and serve.

Nutrition: Calories: 189 | Total Carbs: 2 g | Cholesterol: 13 mg | Total Fats: 7 g | Fiber: 2 g | Protein: 10 g

Provencal Summer Salad

Ingredients:
- 1 zucchini, sliced
- 1 eggplant, sliced
- 2 red onions, sliced
- 2 tomatoes, sliced
- 1 teaspoon dried mint
- 2 garlic cloves, minced
- 2 tablespoons balsamic vinegar
- Salt and pepper to taste

Preparation: 5 min | **Cooking:** 25 min | **Servings:** 2

Directions:
1. Season the zucchini, eggplant, onions, and tomatoes with salt and pepper.
2. Cook the vegetable slices on the grill until browned.
3. Transfer the vegetables to a salad bowl, then add the mint, garlic, and vinegar.
4. Serve the salad right away.

Nutrition: Calories: 74 | Fats: 0.5 g | Protein: 3.0 g | Carbs: 16.5 g

Bean and Toasted Pita Salad

Ingredients:
- 3 tablespoons chopped fresh mint
- 3 tablespoons chopped fresh parsley
- 1 cup crumbled feta cheese
- 1 cup sliced romaine lettuce
- ½ cucumber, peeled and sliced
- 1 cup diced plum tomatoes
- 2 cups cooked pinto beans, well-drained and slightly warmed
- Pepper to taste
- 3 tablespoons extra-virgin olive oil
- 2 tablespoons ground toasted cumin seeds
- 2 tablespoons fresh lemon juice
- 1/8 teaspoon salt
- 2 garlic cloves, peeled
- 2 6-inch whole wheat pita bread, cut or torn into bite-sized pieces

Preparation: 10 min | **Cooking:** 10 min | **Servings:** 4

Directions:
1. On a large baking sheet, spread torn pita bread and bake in a preheated 400F oven for 6 minutes.
2. With the back of a knife, mash garlic and salt until paste-like. Add into a medium bowl.
3. Whisk in ground cumin and lemon juice. In a steady and slow stream, pour oil as you whisk continuously. Season with pepper.
4. In a large salad bowl, mix cucumber, tomatoes, and beans. Pour in dressing, and toss to coat well.
5. Add mint, parsley, feta, lettuce, and toasted pita. Toss to mix once again and serve.

Nutrition: Calories: 427 | Protein: 17.7 g | Carbs: 47.3 g | Fats: 20.4 g

Beans and Spinach Mediterranean Salad

Ingredients:
- 1 can (14 ounces) water-packed artichoke hearts, rinsed, drained, and quartered
- 1 can (14-½ ounces) no-salt-added diced tomatoes, undrained
- 1 can (15 ounces) cannellini beans, rinsed and drained
- 1 small onion, chopped
- 1 tablespoon olive oil
- ¼ teaspoon pepper
- ¼ teaspoon salt
- 1/8 teaspoon crushed red pepper flakes
- 2 garlic cloves, minced
- 2 tablespoons Worcestershire sauce
- 6 ounces fresh baby spinach (about 8 cups)
- Additional olive oil, optional

Preparation: 10 min | **Cooking:** 30 min | **Servings:** 4

Directions:
1. Place a saucepan on medium-high fire and heat for a minute.
2. Add oil and heat for 2 minutes. Stir in onion and sauté for 4 minutes. Add garlic and sauté for another minute.
3. Stir in seasonings, Worcestershire sauce, and tomatoes. Cook for 5 minutes while stirring continuously until the sauce is reduced.
4. Stir in spinach, artichoke hearts, and beans. Sauté for 3 minutes until spinach is wilted and other ingredients are heated through.
5. Serve and enjoy.

Nutrition: Calories: 187 | Protein: 8.0 g | Carbs: 30.0 g | Fats: 4.0 g

Spring Greens Salad

Ingredients:
- ½ cup radish, sliced
- 1 cup fresh spinach, chopped
- ½ cup green peas, cooked
- ½ lemon
- 1 cup arugula, chopped
- 1 tablespoon avocado oil
- ½ teaspoon dried sage

Preparation: 5 min
Cooking: 0 min
Servings: 2

Directions:
1. In the salad bowl, mix up radish, spinach, green peas, arugula, and dried sage.
2. Then squeeze the lemon over the salad.
3. Add avocado oil and shake the salad.

Nutrition: Calories: 54 | Protein: 3.1 g | Carbs: 9 g | Fats: 1.3 g

Tuna Salad

Ingredients:
- ½ cup low-fat Greek yogurt
- 8 ounces tuna, canned
- ½ cup fresh parsley, chopped
- 1 cup corn kernels, cooked
- ½ teaspoon ground black pepper

Preparation: 7 min
Cooking: 0 min
Servings: 2

Directions:
1. Mix up tuna, parsley, kernels, and ground black pepper.
2. Then add yogurt and stir the salad until it is homogenous.

Nutrition: Calories: 172 | Protein: 17.8 g | Carbs: 13.6 g | Fats: 5.5 g

Fish Salad

Ingredients:
- 7 ounces canned salmon, shredded
- 1 tablespoon lime juice
- 1 tablespoon low-fat yogurt
- 1 cup baby spinach, chopped
- 1 teaspoon capers, drained and chopped

Preparation: 5 min
Cooking: 0 min
Servings: 2

Directions:
1. Mix up all ingredients together and transfer them to the salad bowl.

Nutrition: Calories: 71 | Protein: 10.1 g | Carbs: 0.8 g | Fats: 3.2 g

Salmon Salad

Ingredients:
- 4 ounces canned salmon, flaked
- 1 tablespoon lemon juice
- 2 tablespoons red bell pepper, chopped
- 1 tablespoon red onion, chopped
- 1 teaspoon dill, chopped
- 1 tablespoon olive oil

Preparation: 10 min | **Cooking:** 0 min | **Servings:** 2

Directions:
1. Mix up all ingredients in the salad bowl.

Nutrition: Calories: 119 | Protein: 8.3 g | Carbs: 6.6 g | Fats: 7.3 g

Arugula Salad with Shallot

Ingredients:
- 1 cup cucumber, chopped
- 1 tablespoon lemon juice
- 1 tablespoon avocado oil
- 2 shallots, chopped
- ½ cup black olives, sliced
- 3 cups arugula, chopped

Preparation: 10 min | **Cooking:** 0 min | **Servings:** 2

Directions:
1. Mix up all ingredients from the list above in the salad bowl and refrigerate in the fridge for 5 minutes.

Nutrition: Calories: 33 | Protein: 0.8 g | Carbs: 2.9 g | Fat: 2.4 g

Roasted Bell Pepper Salad with Anchovy Dressing

Ingredients:
- 8 roasted red bell peppers, sliced
- 2 tablespoons pine nuts
- 1 cup cherry tomatoes, halved
- 2 tablespoons chopped parsley
- 4 anchovy fillets
- 1 lemon, juiced
- 1 garlic clove
- 1 tablespoon extra-virgin olive oil
- Salt and pepper to taste

Preparation: 10 min | **Cooking:** 20 min | **Servings:** 2

Directions:
1. Combine the anchovy fillets, lemon juice, garlic, and olive oil in a mortar and mix them well.
2. Mix the rest of the ingredients in a salad bowl; then drizzle in the dressing.
3. Serve the salad as fresh as possible.

Nutrition: Calories: 81 | Fats: 7.0 g | Protein: 2.4 g | Carbs: 4.0 g

Roasted Vegetable Salad

Ingredients:
- ½ pound baby carrots
- 2 red onions, sliced
- 1 zucchini, sliced
- 2 eggplants, cubed
- 1 cauliflower, cut into florets
- 1 sweet potato, peeled and cubed
- 1 endive, sliced
- 3 tablespoons extra virgin olive oil
- 1 teaspoon dried basil
- Salt and pepper to taste
- 1 lemon, juiced
- 1 tablespoon balsamic vinegar

Preparation: 0 min
Cooking: 6 min
Servings: 30

Directions:
1. Combine the vegetables with the oil, basil, salt, and pepper in a deep-dish baking pan and cook in a preheated oven at 350°F for 25-30 minutes.
2. When done, transfer to a salad bowl and add the lemon juice and vinegar.
3. Serve the salad fresh.

Nutrition: Calories: 164 | Fats: 7.6 g | Protein: 3.7 g | Carbs: 24.2 g

Spanish Tomato Salad

Ingredients:
- 1-pound tomatoes, cubed
- 2 cucumbers, cubed
- 2 garlic cloves, chopped
- 1 red onion, sliced
- 2 anchovy fillets
- 1 tablespoon balsamic vinegar
- 1 pinch chili powder
- Salt and pepper to taste

Preparation: 5 min
Cooking: 10 min
Servings: 2

Directions:
1. Combine the tomatoes, cucumbers, garlic, and red onion in a bowl.
2. In a mortar, mix the anchovy fillets, vinegar, chili powder, salt, and pepper.
3. Drizzle the mixture over the salad and mix well.
4. Serve the salad fresh.

Nutrition: Calories: 61 | Fats: 0.6 g | Protein: 3.0 g | Carbs: 13.0 g

Grilled Salmon Summer Salad

Ingredients:
- 2 salmon fillets
- Salt and pepper to taste
- 2 cups vegetable stock
- 1 - 2 cups bulgur
- 1 cup cherry tomatoes, halved
- 1 - 2 cups sweet corn
- 1 lemon, juiced
- 1 - 2 cups green olives, sliced
- 1 cucumber, cubed
- 1 green onion, chopped
- 1 red pepper, chopped
- 1 red bell pepper, cored and diced

Preparation: 5 min
Cooking: 30 min
Servings: 2

Directions:
1. Heat a grill pan on medium fire and then place the salmon on, seasoning with salt and pepper. Grill both sides of salmon until brown and set aside.
2. Heat stock in a saucepan until hot. Add in bulgur and cook until liquid is completely soaked into bulgur.
3. Mix salmon, bulgur, and all the other ingredients in a salad bowl. Again, add salt and pepper, if desired, to suit your taste.
4. Serve the salad as soon as completed.

Nutrition: Calories: 69 | Fats: 6.5 g | Carbs: 10.6 g | Protein: 9.4 g

Garden Salad With Oranges and Olives

Ingredients:
- ½ cup red wine vinegar
- 1 tablespoon extra-virgin olive oil
- 1 tablespoon finely chopped celery
- 1 tablespoon finely chopped red onion
- 16 large ripe black olives
- 2 garlic cloves
- 2 navel oranges, peeled and segmented
- 4 boneless, skinless chicken breasts, 4 ounces each
- 4 garlic cloves, minced
- 8 cups leaf lettuce, washed and dried
- Cracked black pepper to taste

Preparation: 5 min
Cooking: 10 min
Servings: 2

Directions:
1. Prepare the dressing by mixing the pepper, celery, onion, olive oil, garlic, and vinegar in a small bowl. Whisk well to combine.
2. Lightly grease a grate and preheat the grill to high.
3. Rub the chicken with the garlic cloves and discard the garlic.
4. Grill the chicken for 5 minutes per side or until cooked through.
5. Remove the chicken from the grill and let it stand for 5 minutes before cutting it into ½-inch strips.
6. On four serving plates, evenly arrange two cups of lettuce, ¼ of the sliced oranges, and 4 olives per plate.
7. Top each plate with ¼ serving of grilled chicken. Evenly drizzle with dressing, serve and enjoy.

Nutrition: Calories: 259.8 | Protein: 18.9 g | Carbs: 12.9 g | Fats: 1.4 g

Salmon & Arugula Salad

Ingredients:
- ¼ cup red onion, sliced thinly
- 1 ½ tablespoon fresh lemon juice
- 1 ½ tablespoon olive oil
- 1 tablespoon extra-virgin olive oil
- 1 tablespoon red wine vinegar
- 2 center-cut salmon fillets (6 ounces each)
- 2/3 cup cherry tomatoes, halved
- 3 cups baby arugula leaves
- Pepper and salt to taste

Preparation: 5 min
Cooking: 10 min
Servings: 2

Directions:
1. In a shallow bowl, mix pepper, salt, 1 ½ tablespoon of olive oil, and lemon juice.
2. Toss in salmon fillets and rub with the marinade. Allow marinating for at least 15 minutes.
3. Grease a baking sheet and preheat the oven to 350°F.
4. Bake the marinated salmon fillet for 10 to 12 minutes or until flaky with the skin side touching the baking sheet.
5. Meanwhile, in a salad bowl mix onion, tomatoes, and arugula.
6. Season with pepper and salt. Drizzle with vinegar and oil. Toss to combine and serve right away with baked salmon on the side.

Nutrition: Calories: 400 | Protein: 26.6 g | Carbs: 5.8 g | Fats: 15.6 g

Farro Salad

Ingredients:
- 1 cup farro
- 1 bay leaf
- 1 shallot
- ¼ cup olive oil
- 1 tablespoon apple cider vinegar
- 1 teaspoon honey
- 1 cup arugula
- 1 apple
- ¼ cup basil
- ¼ cup parsley

Preparation: 5 min
Cooking: 10 min
Servings: 2

Directions:
1. In a bowl, combine all ingredients and mix well.
2. Add dressing and serve.

Nutrition: Calories: 74 | Fats: 7.3 g | Carbs: 12.8 g | Protein: 6.4 g

Carrot Salad

Ingredients:
- 1 lb. carrots
- 1 cup raisins
- ½ cup peanuts
- ½ cup cilantro
- 2 green onions
- ¼ cup olive oil
- 1 tablespoon honey
- 2 garlic cloves
- 1 teaspoon cumin

Preparation: 5 min
Cooking: 10 min
Servings: 2

Directions:
1. In a bowl, combine all ingredients and mix well.
2. Add dressing and serve.

Nutrition: Calories: 69 | Fats: 6.5 g | Carbs: 10.2 g | Protein: 9.4 g

Beets Steamed Edamame Salad

Ingredients:
- 2 bags steamed edamame beans
- White vinegar
- 20-24 ounces can beets
- 4 teaspoons high-quality olive oil
- 12 large organic carrots, cubed
- 6 corns on the cobs, corn cut off
- Black pepper
- 1-pound green beans cut into 1-inch segments

Preparation: 15 min
Cooking: 5 min
Servings: 8

Directions:
1. Wet a paper towel and wrap the corn with the damp towel; place the wrapped corn in the microwave for 5 minutes.
2. Steam the entire ingredients (reserving corn and beets) in a large steamer in this order; carrots cubes, green beans, and edamame beans on the top layer.
3. Mix beets together with the cooked corn and cooked vegetables.
4. Toss salad slightly with a few dashes of black pepper, white vinegar, and olive oil.

Nutrition: Calories: 317 | Fats: 16.5 g | Carbs: 17.6 g | Protein: 12.4 g

Avocado Cilantro Chunky Salsa

Ingredients:
- 6 tablespoons chopped cilantro leaves
- 3 tablespoons avocado or macadamia nut oil
- 3 large diced ripe tomato
- 1 ½ finely diced spring onion
- 3 large diced avocados
- Salt and pepper
- 6 tablespoons lime juice

Preparation: 10 min
Cooking: 0 min
Servings: 6

Directions:
1. Add all the ingredients to a bowl and carefully toss.
2. Serve right away.

Nutrition: Calories: 350 | Fats: 16.5 g | Carbs: 14.2 g | Protein: 7.4 g

Toasted Mango Pepitas Kale Salad

Ingredients:
- 4 teaspoons honey
- 2 fresh mangos, thinly diced (about 1 cup)
- Freshly ground black pepper
- 4 tablespoons toasted pepitas
- Kosher salt
- 1 lemon juice
- 2 large bunch kale de-stalk and sliced into ribbons
- ½ cup extra-virgin olive oil, plus more

Preparation: 20 min
Cooking: 0 min
Servings: 8

Directions:
1. Add the sliced kale into a large mixing bowl; add half the lemon juice and little salt.
2. Start working on the kale using your fingertips for 5 minutes or until the kale leaves are tender and sweet.
3. Spread olive oil over the kale and work on the kale with your finger for a few more minutes. Set aside.
4. Blend the black pepper and honey with the remaining half lemon juice in a small bowl.
5. Steadily drip in ½ cup of olive oil while whisking until it forms a dressing. Season dressing with a pinch of salt.
6. Pour a few dressings on the kale and add the pepitas and mango. Toss together and serve.

Nutrition: Calories: 158 | Fats: 6.5 g | Carbs: 5.6 g | Protein: 6.2 g

Chickpeas and Parsley Pumpkin Salad

Ingredients:
- 1 ½ small thinly sliced red onion
- 1 ½ handful parsley, chopped
- 1 ½ diced avocado
- 1 ½ tablespoons lemon juice
- 1 ½ teaspoons ground coriander
- 1 ½ teaspoons ground cumin
- Salt and pepper to season
- 3 tablespoons olive oil
- 1 ½ cup pumpkin, peeled and chopped into bite pieces
- 1 ½ (21.5 ounces) can chickpeas, rinsed and drained

Preparation: 5 min

Cooking: 10 min

Servings: 6

Directions:
1. Season the pumpkin with a drizzle of olive oil, coriander, and cumin on top.
2. Arrange seasoned pumpkin in an oven tray lined with parchment paper.
3. Roast until the pumpkin is lightly browned and soft.
4. Combine the salad ingredients in a bowl and drizzle in lemon juice.

Nutrition: Calories: 113 | Fats: 7 g | Carbs: 4.8 g | Protein: 11.4 g

Springtime Chicken Berries Salad

Ingredients:
Salad:
- 4 cups quartered strawberries
- 2/3 cup vertically sliced red onion
- 2 cups fresh blueberries
- 24 ounces boneless, skinless, rotisserie chicken breast, sliced
- 8 cups arugula
- 8 cups torn romaine lettuce

Dressing:
- 2 tablespoons water
- 2/8 teaspoon freshly ground black pepper
- 2/8 teaspoon salt
- 4 tablespoons extra-virgin olive oil
- 4 tablespoons red wine vinegar
- 2 tablespoons of low-carb sweetener of your choice

Preparation: 5 min

Cooking: 5 min

Servings: 8

Directions:
1. In a large mixing bowl, combine the blueberries, strawberries, arugula, romaine, and onions. Toss gently to combine.
2. In a small bowl, combine 2 tablespoons of water, black pepper, red wine vinegar, salt, and sweetener. Fold in the olive oil, stirring often until well incorporated.
3. Arrange eight different plates and place up to 2 cups of chicken mixture on each. Drizzle with four teaspoons of the dressing.

Nutrition: Calories: 317 | Fats: 9.5 g | Carbs: 16.7 g | Protein: 18.2 g

Toaster Almond Spiralized Beet Salad

Ingredients:
- 1/8 teaspoon ground pepper
- 1/8 cup extra-virgin olive oil
- ¼ teaspoon freshly grated lemon zest
- 1-pound beets (2 medium)
- ¼ cup (fresh) chopped flat-leaf parsley
- 1 tablespoon lemon juice
- ¼ cup slivered almonds, toasted
- ¼ teaspoon salt
- 1/6 cup minced shallot

Preparation: 15 min
Cooking: 15 min
Servings: 4

Directions:
1. Mix the minced shallot, lemon juice, oil, salt, pepper, and lemon zest in a small bowl. Mix gently to combine; then set aside.
2. Peel the beets with a thin blade; then spiralize and cut into 3-inch lengths.
3. Arrange the spiralized beets into a large bowl. Sprinkle beets on top with the dressing, and toss gently to make sure the salad is finely coated.
4. Add chopped parsley and almonds before serving. Toss to coat.

Nutrition: Calories: 234 | Fats: 7.8 g | Fiber: 12.6 g | Carbs: 14.6 g | Protein: 8.3 g

Eggplant Garlic Salad with Tomatoes

Ingredients:
- 3 tomatoes, chopped
- 2 eggplants, chopped
- 1 tablespoon olive oil
- 1 teaspoon avocado oil
- 1 tablespoon vinegar
- ½ teaspoon ground black pepper
- ½ teaspoon dried basil
- 2 garlic cloves, chopped

Preparation: 10 min
Cooking: 15 min
Servings: 6

Directions:
1. Place the chopped eggplants in the Air Fryer.
2. Sprinkle the eggplants with olive oil, ground black pepper, and dried basil.
3. Stir the eggplants and cook for 15 minutes at 390F. Stir the vegetables every 5 minutes.
4. Then place the tomatoes in the bowl.
5. Add cooked eggplants, vinegar, and chopped garlic.
6. Next, sprinkle the salad with the avocado oil and stir it.
7. Serve the cooked salad or keep it in the fridge!

Nutrition: Calories: 80 | Fats: 2.9 | Carbs: 13.6 | Protein: 2.4

Chapter 11

Desserts

Honey-Cinnamon Grilled Plums

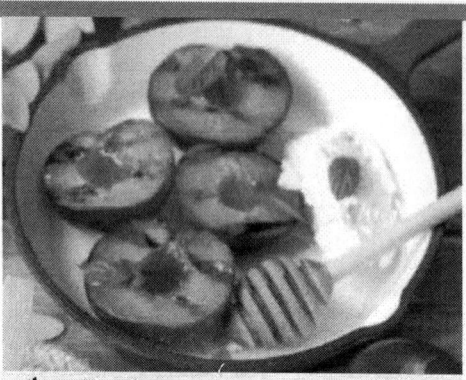

Preparation: 15 min

Cooking: 5 min

Servings: 4

Direction

1. Preheat the grill to medium heat.
2. Brush the plum halves with olive oil. Grill, flesh-side down, for 4 to 5 minutes, then flip and cook for another 4 to 5 minutes, until just tender.
3. In a small bowl, whisk together the honey and cinnamon.
4. Scoop the frozen yogurt into 4 bowls. Place 2 plum halves in each bowl and drizzle each with the cinnamon-honey mixture.

NUTRITION: 193 calories 8g fat 3g protein 30g carbohydrates 62mg

Ingredients:

- 4 large plums, sliced in half and pitted
- 1 tablespoon olive oil
- 1 tablespoon honey
- 1 teaspoon ground cinnamon
- 2 cups vanilla bean frozen yogurt

Lemon Ricotta Peaches

Ingredients:

- 6 ripe peaches, pitted and thinly sliced
- ¼ cup water
- 2 tablespoons of raw sugar
- 1½ tablespoons lemon juice
- 1 cup low-fat ricotta
- 2 teaspoons lemon zest

Direction

1. In a heavy, medium-sized skillet, combine peaches, water, sugar, and lemon juice. Bring just to a simmer, stirring frequently. Remove from heat.
2. In a small bowl, combine ricotta and lemon zest. Mix well.
3. Divide peaches between four bowls. Top with ricotta and serve.

NUTRITION: 166 calories 5.3g fat 8g protein 26g carbohydrates

Rhubarb Compote

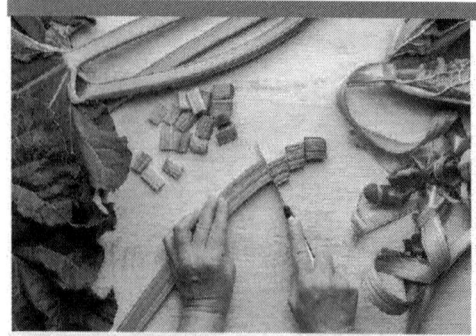

Preparation: 10 min

Cooking: 15 min

Servings: 4

Directions:

1. In a pot, combine the rhubarb with the other ingredients, toss, bring to a boil over medium heat, cook for 15 minutes, divide into bowls and serve cold.

NUTRITION: 52 calories 0.6g protein 11.9g carbohydrates 0.1g fat

Ingredients:

- 2 cups rhubarb, roughly chopped
- 3 tablespoons coconut sugar
- 1 teaspoon almond extract
- 2 cups of water

Grilled Pineapple Strips

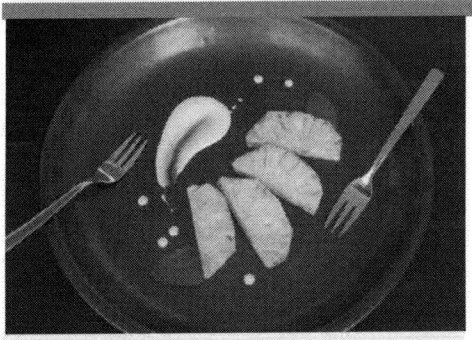

Ingredients:
- Sunflower oil
- Dash of iodized salt
- 1 pineapple
- 1 tablespoon lime juice extract
- 1 tablespoon olive oil
- 1 tablespoon raw honey
- 3 tablespoons brown sugar

Directions:
1. Peel the pineapple, remove the eyes of the fruit, and discard the core. Slice lengthwise, forming six wedges. Mix the rest of the fixing in a bowl until blended.
2. Brush the coating mixture on the pineapple (reserve some for basting). Grease an oven or outdoor grill rack with the oil.
3. Place the pineapple wedges on the grill rack and heat for a few minutes per side until golden brownish, basting it frequently with a reserved glaze. Serve on a platter.

NUTRITION: Calories 87 Fats 2 g Carbohydrates 20 g Fibers 1 g Proteins 1 g

Nutmeg Lemon Pudding

Ingredients:
- 2 tablespoons lemon marmalade
- 4 eggs, whisked
- 2 tablespoons stevia
- 3 cups almond milk
- 4 allspice berries, crushed
- ¼ teaspoon nutmeg, grated

Preparation: 5 min
Cooking: 20 min
Servings: 2

Directions:
1. In a bowl, mix the lemon marmalade with the eggs and the other ingredients and whisk well.
2. Divide the mix into ramekins, introduce in the oven and bake at 350 degrees F for 20 minutes.
3. Serve cold.

Nutrition: calories 220, fat 6.6, fiber 3.4, carbs 12.4, protein 3.4

Fruit Medley

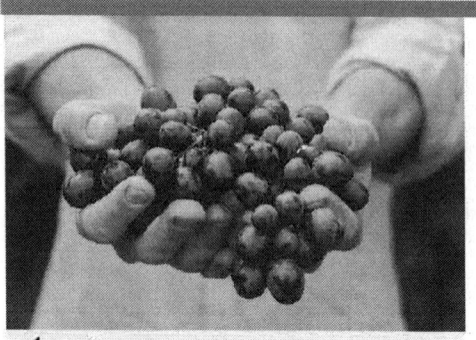

Preparation: 5 min
Cooking: 10 min
Servings: 7

Ingredients:
- 4 fuyu persimmons, sliced into wedges
- 1 ½ cups grapes, halved
- 8 mint leaves, chopped
- 1 tablespoon lemon juice
- 1 tablespoon honey
- ½ cups almond, toasted and chopped

Directions:
1. Combine all Ingredients: in a bowl.
2. Toss then chill before serving.

Nutrition: Calories per serving:159; Carbs: 32g; Protein: 3g; Fat: 4g

Lemon and Semolina Cookies

Ingredients:
- ½ teaspoon lemon zest, grated
- 4 tablespoons semolina
- 2 tablespoons olive oil
- 8 tablespoons wheat flour, whole grain
- 1 teaspoon vanilla extract
- ½ teaspoon ground clove
- 3 tablespoons coconut oil
- ¼ teaspoon baking powder
- ¼ cup of water

Preparation: 5 min
Cooking: 20 min
Servings: 2

Directions:
1. Make the dough: in the mixing bowl combine together lemon zest, semolina, olive oil, wheat flour, vanilla extract, ground clove, coconut oil, and baking powder.
2. Knead the soft dough.
3. Make the small cookies in the shape of walnuts and press them gently with the help of the fork.
4. Line the baking tray with the baking paper.
5. Place the cookies in the tray and bake them for 20 minutes at 375F.
6. Meanwhile, bring the water to boil.
7. Pour the cooled sweet water over the hot baked cookies and leave them for 10 minutes.
8. When the cookies soak all liquid, transfer them in the serving plates.

Nutrition: calories 165, fat 11.7, fiber 0.6, carbs 23.7, protein 2

Semolina Cake

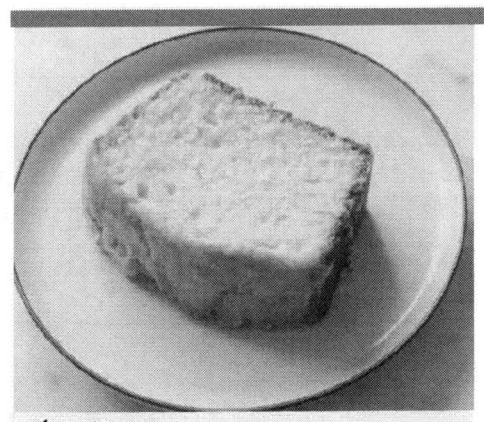

Preparation: 5 min
Cooking: 20 min
Servings: 6

Directions:

1. Mix up together wheat flour, semolina, baking powder, Plain yogurt, vanilla extract and olive oil.
2. Then add lemon rind and mix up the ingredients until smooth.
3. Transfer the mixture in the non-sticky cake mold, sprinkle with almond flakes, and bake for 30 minutes at 365F.
4. Meanwhile, bring the orange juice to boil.
5. Add liquid honey and stir until dissolved.
6. When the cake is cooked, pour the hot orange juice mixture over it and let it rest for at least 10 minutes.
7. Cut the cake into the servings.

Nutrition: calories 179, fat 6.1, fiber 1.1, carbs 36.3, protein 4.5

Ingredients:

- ½ cup wheat flour, whole grain
- ½ cup semolina
- 1 teaspoon baking powder
- ½ cup Plain yogurt
- 1 teaspoon vanilla extract
- 1 teaspoon lemon rind
- 2 tablespoons olive oil
- 1 tablespoon almond flakes
- 4 teaspoons liquid honey
- ½ cup of orange juice

Banana Kale Smoothie

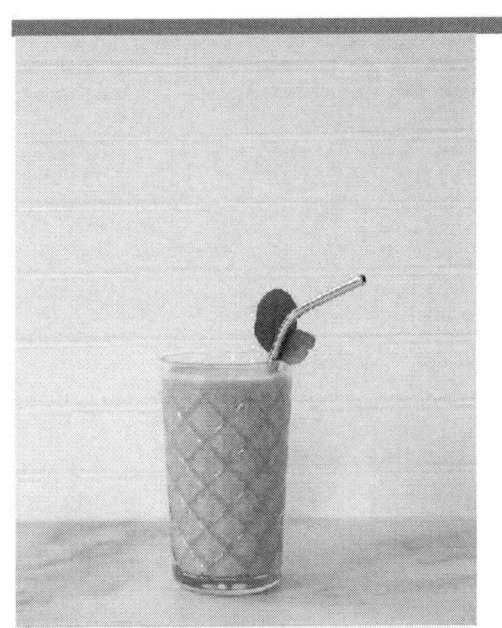

Preparation: 5 min
Cooking: 10 min
Servings: 2

Directions:

1. Place all Ingredients: in a blender.
2. Blend until smooth.
3. Pour in a glass container and allow to chill in the fridge for at least 30 minutes.

Nutrition: Calories per serving: 165; Carbs: 32.1g; Protein: 2.3g; Fat: 4.2g

Ingredients:

- 2 cups kale leaves
- 1 cup almond milk
- ½ cup crushed ice
- 1 banana, peeled
- 1 apple, peeled and cored
- A dash of cinnamon

Lime Grapes and Apples

Ingredients:
- ½ cup red grapes
- 2 apples
- 1 teaspoon lime juice
- 1 teaspoon Erythritol
- 3 tablespoons water

Preparation: 5 min
Cooking: 25 min
Servings: 2

Directions:
1. Line the baking tray with baking paper.
2. Then cut the apples on the halves and remove the seeds with the help of the scooper.
3. Cut the apple halves on 2 parts more.
4. Arrange all fruits in the tray in one layer, drizzle with water, and bake for 20 minutes at 375F.
5. Flip the fruits on another side after 10 minutes of cooking.
6. Then remove them from the oven and sprinkle with lime juice and Erythritol.
7. Return the fruits back in the oven and bake for 5 minutes more.
8. Serve the cooked dessert hot or warm.

Nutrition: calories 142, fat 0.4, fiber 5.7, carbs 40.1, protein 0.9

Apple Crisp

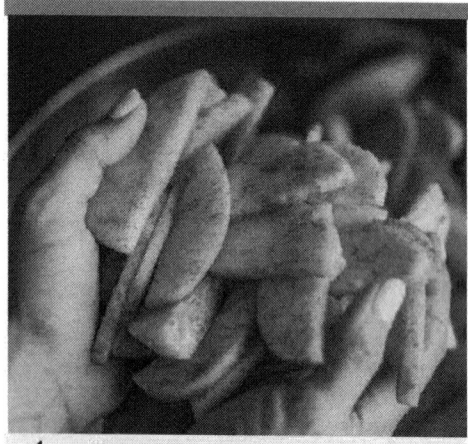

Preparation: 5 min
Cooking: 10 min
Servings: 2

Directions
1. Preheat the oven to 300 degrees F.
2. In a large baking dish, place all filling ingredients and gently mix.
3. In a bowl, mix together all topping ingredients.
4. Spread the topping over filling mixture evenly.
5. Bake for about 20 minutes or until top becomes golden brown.

Nutrition: Calories 185, Fat 6.5 g, Fiber 0.6 g, Carbs 22.6 g, Protein 4.4 g

Ingredients
- For Filling
- 2 large apples, peeled, cored and chopped
- 2 tbsp. fresh apple juice
- 2 tbsp. water
- ¼ tsp. ground cinnamon
- For Topping
- ½ C. quick rolled oats
- ¼ C. unsweetened coconut flakes
- 2 tbsp. walnuts, chopped
- ½ tsp. ground cinnamon
- ¼ C. water

Strawberry and Avocado Medley

Ingredients:
- 2 cups strawberry, halved
- 1 avocado, pitted and sliced
- 2 tablespoons slivered almonds

Preparation: 5 min
Cooking: 10 min
Servings: 2

Directions:
1. Place all Ingredients: in a mixing bowl.
2. Toss to combine.
3. Allow to chill in the fridge before serving.

Nutrition: Calories per serving: 107; Carbs: 9.9g; Protein: 1.6g; Fat: 7.8g

Watermelon Ice Cream

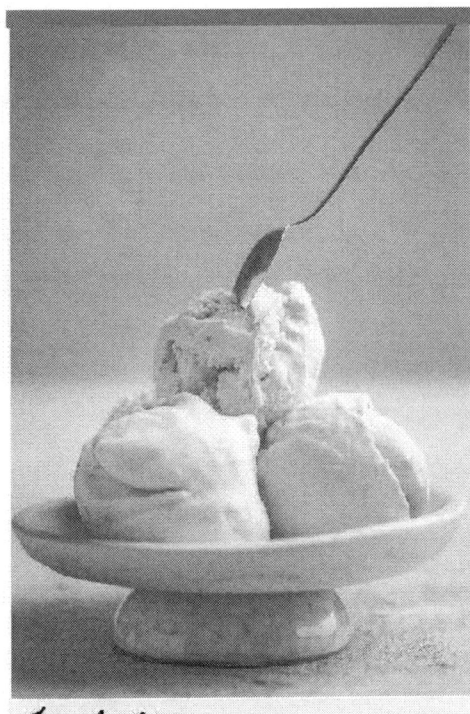

Preparation: 5 min
Cooking: 10 min
Servings: 2

Directions:
1. Make the juice from the watermelon with the help of the fruit juices.
2. Combine together 5 tablespoons of watermelon juice and 1 tablespoon of gelatin powder. Stir it and leave for 5 minutes.
3. Then preheat the watermelon juice until warm, add gelatin mixture and heat it up over the medium heat until gelatin is dissolved.
4. Then remove the liquid from the heat and put it in the silicone molds.
5. Freeze the jelly for 30 minutes in the freezer or for 4 hours in the fridge.

Nutrition: calories 46, fat 0.2, fiber 0.4, carbs 8.5, protein 3.7

Ingredients:
- 8 oz watermelon
- 1 tablespoon gelatin powder

Raspberry Walnut Sorbet

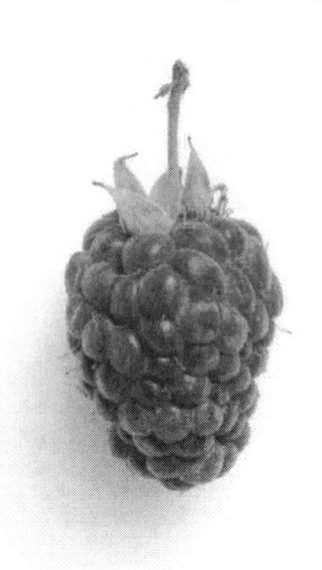

Preparation: 5 min

Cooking: 0 min

Servings: 4

Direction

1. In a food processor or blender, purée all ingredients together. Freeze in an ice cream maker. Alternately, spread fruit mixture onto a cookie sheet and place in freezer.
2. Every 20 minutes, scrape through fruit mixture with a spoon so that it doesn't freeze into a solid mass (this will keep it nice and light).

Nutrition 75 calories 4g fat 2g protein 9g carbohydrates

Ingredients:

- 2 cups fresh ripe raspberries
- ¼ cup chopped walnuts
- 1 teaspoon lemon juice
- 2 tablespoons organic agave nectar

Juices & Smoothies

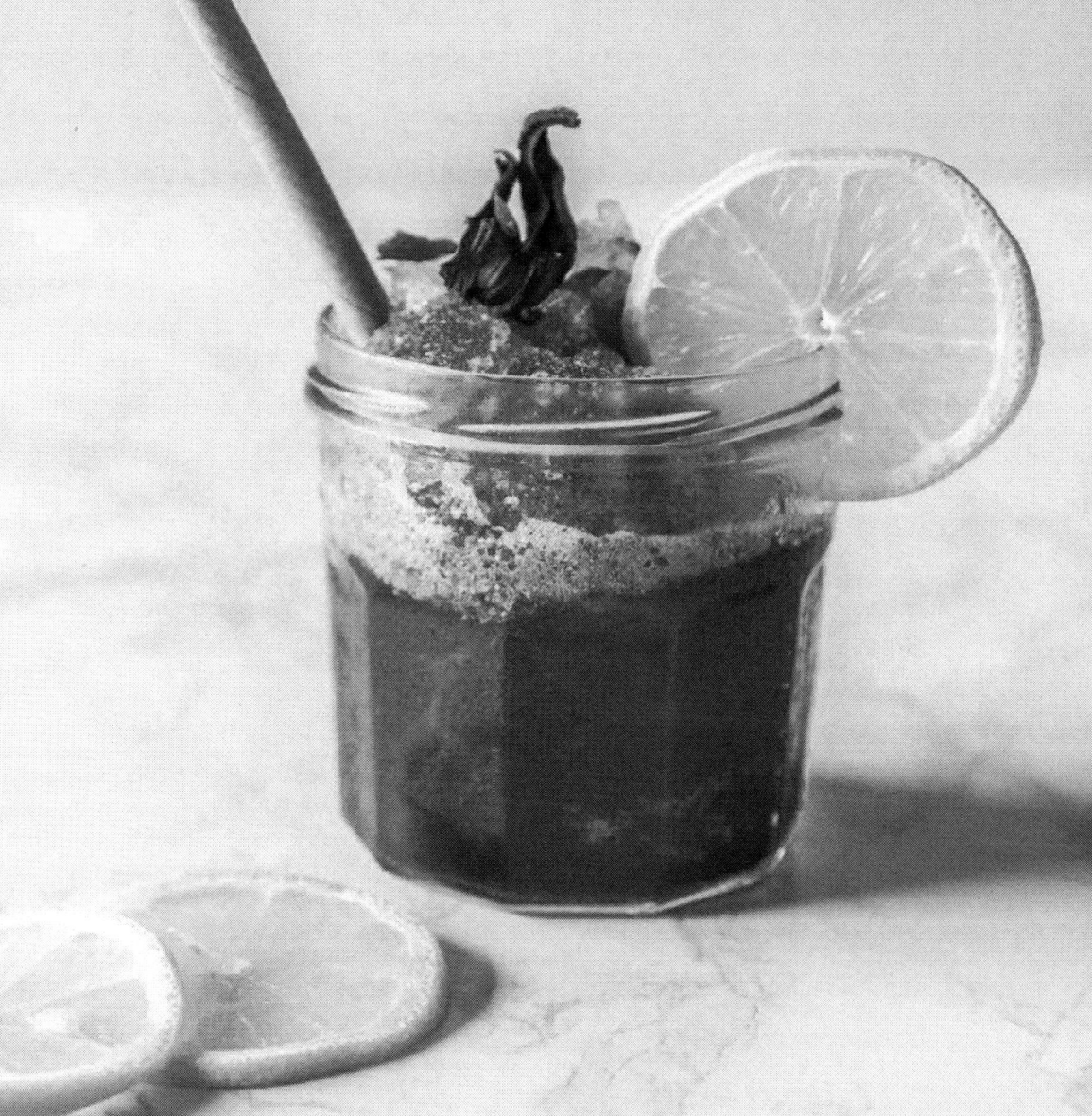

Chapter 12

Breakfast Smoothie

Ingredients:
- Frozen blueberries – 1 cup
- Pineapple chunks – ½ cup
- English cucumber – ½ cup
- Apple – ½
- Water – ½ cup

Preparation: 15 min

Cooking: 0 min

Servings: 2

Directions:
1. Put the pineapple, blueberries, cucumber, apple, and water in a blender and blend until thick and smooth.
2. Pour into 2 glasses and serve.

NUTRITION: Calories: 87 Fat: g Carb: 22g Protein: 0.7g

Clean Liver Green Juice

Ingredients
- 2½ C. fresh spinach
- 2 large celery stalks
- 2 large green apples, cored and sliced
- 1 medium orange, peeled, seeded and sectioned
- 1 tbsp. fresh lime juice
- 1 tbsp. fresh lemon juice

Preparation: 10 min

Cooking: 0 min

Servings: 2

Directions
1. In a juicer, add all ingredients and extract the juice according to manufacturer's directions.
2. Transfer into 2 serving glasses and stir in lime and lemon juices.
3. Serve immediately.

Nutrition: Calories 110, Fat 3, Fiber 9, Carbs 25, Protein 4

Green Tea Purifying Smoothie

Ingredients
- 2 C. fresh baby spinach
- 3 C. frozen green grapes
- 1 medium ripe avocado peeled, pitted and chopped
- 2 tsp. organic honey
- 1½ C. strong brewed green tea

Preparation: 10 min

Cooking: 0 min

Servings: 2

Directions
1. a high-speed blender, add all ingredients and pulse until smooth.
2. Transfer into serving glasses and serve immediately.

Nutrition: Calories 138, Fat 3, Fiber 8, Carbs 28, Protein 3

Blue Breeze Shake

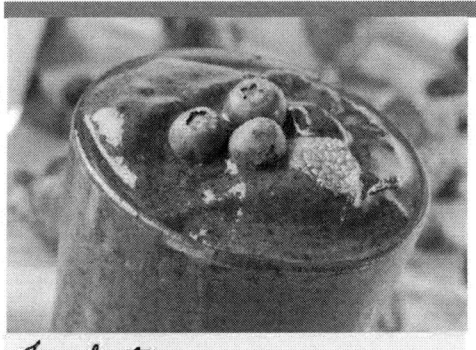

Preparation: 10 min

Cooking: 0 min

Servings: 2

Ingredients:
- ½ cup blueberries
- 1 small banana
- 1 cup chilled unsweetened vanilla almond milk
- Water as needed
- 1 scoop unflavored protein powder

Directions:
1. Mix in a blender for 40-50 seconds and serve as ready.

Nutrition: Calories 220, Fat 40, Carbs 48, Protein 5.5

Fats Burning & Water Based Smoothies

Ingredients:
- ¾ cup water
- Ice as needed
- 4 big strawberries
- 1 small piece of banana or an apple slice with peel
- ¼ teaspoon of cinnamon powder
- 1 teaspoon honey

Preparation: 10 min

Cooking: 0 min

Servings: 2

Directions:
1. Take a blender and add water, remove stems from the berries and add in the blender, put cinnamon powder, honey, crushed ice cubes and remaining fruit. Mix and serve.

Nutrition: Calories 170, Fat 2, Carbs 12, Protein 5

Smoothie with Ginger and Cucumber

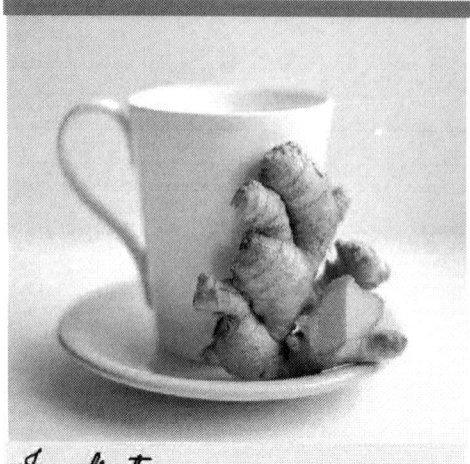

Preparation: 10 min **Cooking:** 0 min **Servings:** 2

Directions:

1. Add chilled cup of water in an electric mixer, grate ginger piece. Mix with cucumber slices, lime juice and mint leaves to serve.

Nutrition: Calories 80, Fat 1, Carbs 8, Protein 3

Ingredients:

- 1 cup chilled water
- 2 slices of cucumber
- 1 tablespoon lime juice
- Couple of mint leaves
- 1 small piece of ginger fresh

Oatmeal Blast with Fruit

Ingredients:

- ½ cup oats (steel cut)
- A pinch of ground cinnamon
- Ice cubes as needed
- 1 cup water
- ½ cup pineapple chunks

Preparation: 10 min **Cooking:** 0 min **Servings:** 2

Directions:

1. Throw oats in a blender and slightly blend with water, add the fruit and other ingredients afterwards and blend again.

Nutrition: Calories 160, Fat 1, Carbs 18, Protein 4

White Bean Smoothie to Burn Fats

Ingredients:

- 1 cup unsweetened rice milk (chilled)
- ¼ cup peach slices
- ¼ cup white beans cooked
- A pinch of cinnamon powder
- A pinch of nutmeg

Preparation: 10 min **Cooking:** 0 min **Servings:** 2

Directions:

1. Pour milk in the blender and add other ingredients to blend till smooth enough to serve and drink.

Nutrition: Calories 335, Fat 3, Carbs 28, Protein 9

Meal Replacement Smoothie with Banana

Ingredients:
- 1 large banana (ripped or green)
- 1 cup coconut milk
- A drop of vanilla extract
- 1 tablespoon of natural peanut powder
- 1 teaspoon carob powder
- Ice as needed
- 4 small fresh berries without stems

Preparation: 10 min **Cooking:** 0 min **Servings:** 2

Directions:
1. Mix all foods and condiments in milk and shake them all well in an electric machine.

Nutrition: Calories 330, Fat 28, Carbs 14, Protein 11

Coconut Cherry Smoothie

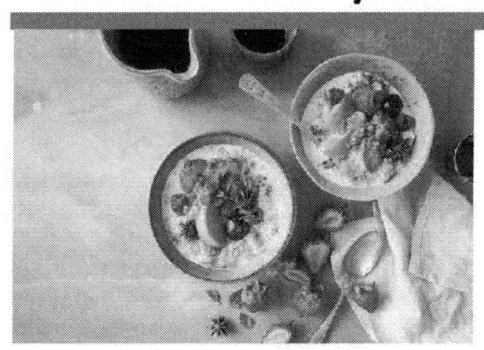

Preparation: 10 min **Cooking:** 0 min **Servings:** 2

Directions:
1. Toss in the berries, milk and other ingredients in a blender, shake well to make a smooth drink.

Nutrition: Calories 220, Fat 24, Carbs 11, Protein 6

Ingredients:
- 1 cup coconut milk
- 4 Ice cubes as needed
- 1 cup mixed berries (blueberries, blackberries and cherries)
- ½ plantains
- A handful of mixed chopped fruits- pear/peach/guava/strawberry
- 2 tablespoons plain soy yogurt

Grapes and Peach Smoothie

Ingredients:
- 1 cup red grapes juice
- 3 tablespoon shredded coconut
- ½ scoop protein powder
- A handful of chopped pistachios
- 1 small guava and peach chopped
- Ice as required

Preparation: 10 min **Cooking:** 0 min **Servings:** 2

Directions:
1. Use natural juice to add in the smoothie, mix all the foods in a blender and shake to make it a smooth drink.

Nutrition: Calories 148, Fat 2, Carbs 19, Protein 5

Twin Berry Smoothie

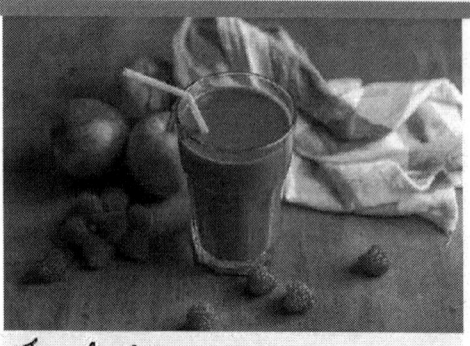

Ingredients:

1. ½ cup peach chunks
2. ¾ cup almond milk
3. A handful of cranberries and raspberries
4. Peel of an orange
5. 1 scoop protein powder (whey)
6. Ice cubes as required

Directions:

1. Chop berries well, use natural orange peel, add all foods in a blender and shake to serve.

Nutrition: Calories 110, Fat 3, Carbs 7, Protein 18

Light Fiber Smoothie

Ingredients:

- 2 teaspoons nutmeg
- 1 ½ scoop vanilla protein powder mix
- 1½ cup soy milk
- ½ cup low fat egg nog
- A pinch of cinnamon
- 4-5 crushed ice cubes
- 1 lemon zest

Preparation: 10 min

Cooking: 0 min

Servings: 2

Directions:

1. Grab the ingredients, measure and add them all in a blender to mix for a drink.

Nutrition: Calories 160, Fat 8, Carbs 6, Protein 16

Peach and Kiwi Smoothie

Ingredients:

- 1 cup plain low fat yogurt
- ½ cup peach chunks
- 1 tablespoon protein powder
- Water as needed
- ½ cup kiwi fruit

Preparation: 10 min

Cooking: 0 min

Servings: 2

Directions:

1. Blend powder and fruits finely in liquid, serve chilled when smooth.

Nutrition: Calories 130, Fat 3, Carbs 9, Protein 9

Cashew Boost Smoothie

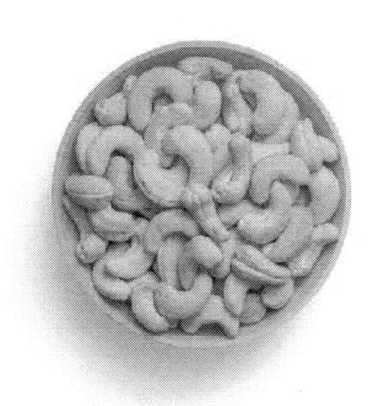

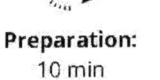

Preparation: 10 min
Cooking: 0 min
Servings: 2

Directions:

1. Grind all ingredients mixed and serve.

Nutrition: Calories 191, Fat 8, Carbs 9, Protein 16

Ingredients:

- 2/4 cup raw cashews
- 1 cup chilled almond milk
- ¼ cup mixed fruit

Heavy Metal Cleansing Smoothie

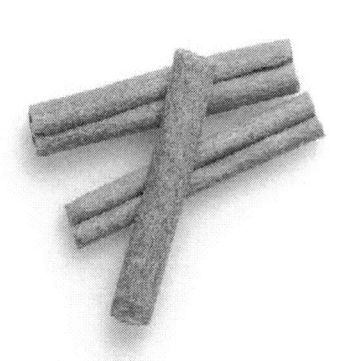

Preparation: 10 min
Cooking: 0 min
Servings: 2

Directions:

1. Take a blender and combine all ingredients to mix and serve when smooth. Serve at room temperature or slightly warm as you like.

Nutrition: Calories 69, Fat 3.5 g, Carbs 10.6 g, Protein 8.4 g

Ingredients:

- 1 cup soy milk
- A pinch of turmeric
- A pinch of freshly crushed ginger
- 1 teaspoon cinnamon powder
- 1 tablespoon maple syrup
- A big date without pit

Power Detox Smoothie

Ingredients:
- 1 table spoon honey
- 1 cup almond milk (unsweetened)
- 1 teaspoon ginger paste
- A pinch of flaxseeds
- ¼ cup cherries without pits
- Ice to chill
- Few drops lemon juice

Preparation: 10 min

Cooking: 0 min

Servings: 2

Directions:
1. Blend milk with cherries first and then add the rest of the ingredients with ice. Serve chilled.

Nutrition: Calories 69, Fat 3.5 g, Carbs 10.6 g, Protein 4.4 g

Detox Action Super Green Smoothie

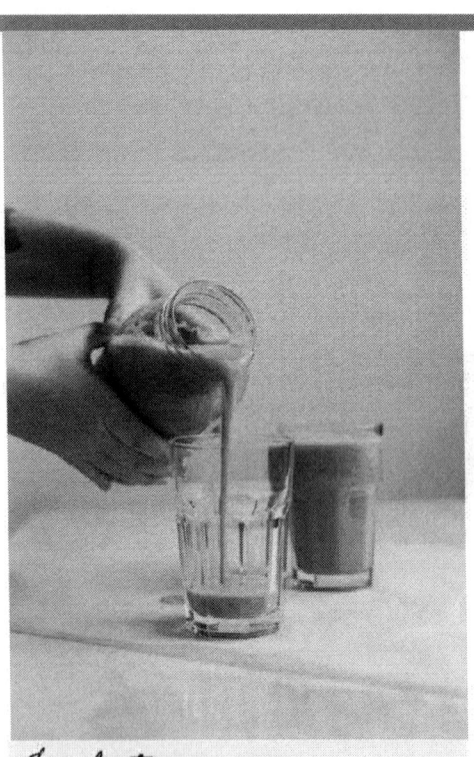

Preparation: 10 min

Cooking: 0 min

Servings: 2

Directions:
1. Blend all the above listed ingredients in an electric blender and serve immediately. Fresh smoothie is the best to consume.

Nutrition: Calories 110, Fat 3.5 g, Carbs 11.2 g, Protein 3.4 g

Ingredients:
- 1 cup chilled mango juice
- ¼ cup chopped flat leaf parsley
- ¼ cup chilled tangerine
- 1 Medium ribs celery
- ½ cup orange pulp without seeds

Kale Batch Detox Smoothie

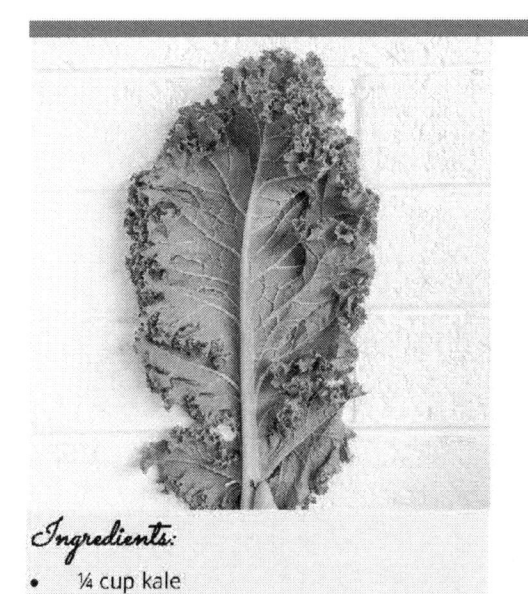

Preparation: 10 min

Cooking: 0 min

Servings: 2

Directions:

1. Blend all the ingredients in a blender for a minute and serve fresh.

   Nutrition: Calories 191, Fat 10, Carbs 13, Protein 2

Ingredients:

- ¼ cup kale
- 1 cup chilled coconut water
- 2 pear slices
- ¼ cup avocado
- A handful of cilantro

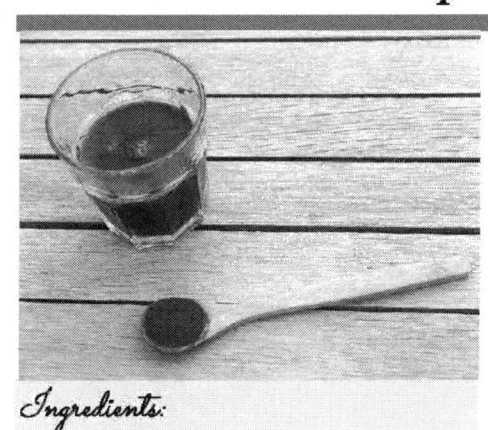

Smoothie with A Spirit

Preparation: 10 min

Cooking: 0 min

Servings: 2

Directions:

1. Mix all the ingredients in a mixing blender and serve as soon as it becomes smooth.

   Nutrition: Calories 169, Fat 3.5 g, Carbs 13.6 g, Protein 6.4 g

Ingredients:

- ¼ cup Greek yogurt
- ½ of a banana
- 1 teaspoon spirulina
- ¼ cup blueberries
- ½ cup chilled almond milk
- ¼ cup peach chunks

Alkaline Green Bliss Smoothie

Ingredients:
- ¼ cup spinach
- ¼ pear slices
- 1 cup chilled water
- A pinch of pumpkin seeds

Preparation: 10 min

Cooking: 0 min

Servings: 2

Preparation

1. Just mix all ingredients in water and transfer in a glass to drink.

Nutrition: Calories 79, Fat 1 g, Carbs 5.2 g, Protein 2.4 g

Smooth Root Green Cleansing Smoothie

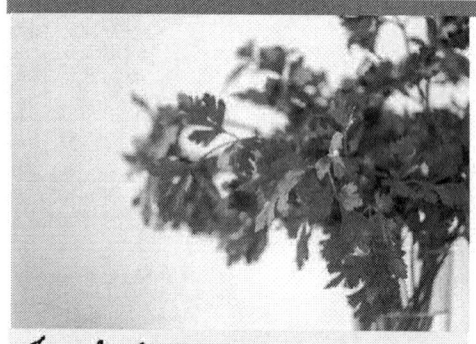

Directions:

1. Wash apple and leaves well before use, do not peel apple just remove seeds and inedible parts, mix all the ingredients blend and serve.

Nutrition: Calories 88, Fat 2, Carbs 7, Protein 4

Ingredients:
- ½ cup fresh lettuce leaves
- ¼ green apple chunks
- A handful of cilantro
- ¼ lime juice
- Couple of cucumber slices
- 1 date without pit
- 1 cup chilled water

Glory Smoothie

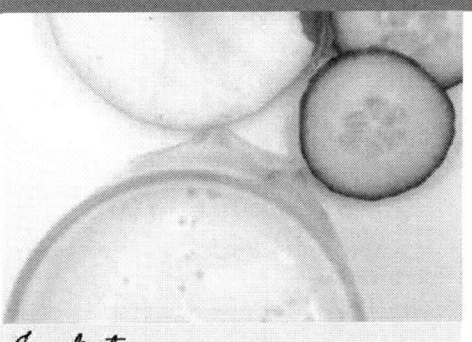

Directions:

1. This smoothie is preparation ared by combining all ingredients listed above with juice and shake well to form a smooth drink to serve. Use ice or chilled juice to get drink chilled.

Nutrition: Calories 113, Fat 2.5 g, Carbs 10.6 g, Protein 6.4 g

Ingredients:

- ¼ cup kale
- A handful of romaine
- A handful of broccoli stems
- A celery stalk
- 1 cup juice of green apple
- 2 big cucumber slices
- ½ of a lemon juice and zest both

Strawberry Nutty Smoothie

Ingredients:

- ½ cup strawberries
- 1 cup nut milk
- 1 tablespoon honey
- 2 slices of orange
- 2 drops of lemon juice
- ½ of a banana slices
- ¼ cup spinach

Preparation: 10 min
Cooking: 0 min
Servings: 2

Directions:

1. You can also use any skimmed milk, remove stems of strawberries and after washing all foods, chop and mix them in a blender to shake and serve in a glass.

Nutrition: Calories 139, Fat 2 g, Carbs 11.6 g, Protein 7.2 g

Tropical Green Tea

Ingredients

- 7 C. boiling water
- ¼ C. fresh ginger, chopped
- 5 green tea bags
- ¼ C. frozen pineapple, peeled and cubed
- ¼ C. frozen mango, peeled, pitted and cubed
- 1 orange, seeded and cut into rings
- 1 lemon, seeded and cut into rings

Preparation: 10 min
Cooking: 0 min
Servings: 2

Directions

1. In a pan, add water and ginger and bring to a boil.
2. Remove from the heat and stir in the tea bags.
3. Cover the pan tightly and steep for about 15 minutes.
4. Through a strainer, strain the mixture into a large glass pitcher.
5. Stir in remaining ingredients and keep aside at the room temperature to cool completely.
6. Refrigerate to chill before serving.

Nutrition: Calories 101, Fat 1, Carbs 10, Protein

Old Spice Ginger Tea

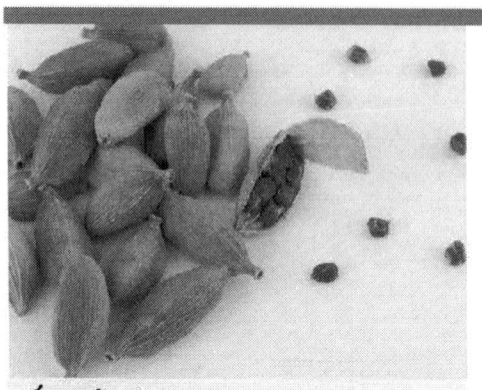

Preparation: 10 min
Cooking: 0 min
Servings: 2

Directions

1. In a pan, add water over medium-high heat and bring to a boil.
2. Add ginger, lemon slices and spices and stir to combine.
3. Reduce the heat to medium-low and simmer for about 5-10 minutes.
4. Through a strainer, strain the tea into a pitcher, discarding the solids.
5. Stir in honey and serve.

Nutrition: Calories 98, Fat 0.5 g, Carbs 15.6 g, Protein 1.4 g

Ingredients

- 8 C. water
- 1 (4-inch) piece fresh ginger, chopped
- 4 lemons, sliced
- 6 cardamom pods, bruised
- 1 cinnamon stick
- 1 whole star anise pod
- 3 tbsp. organic honey

Healthy Vacation Peach Drink

Ingredients:

- 2 fresh lemon juice
- Ice cubes
- 10 tbsp of sweetener of choice
- 5 cups of water
- 8 peeled peaches, cut into slices
- For garnish:
- Mint leaves
- Peach slices

Preparation: 5 min
Cooking: 5 min
Servings: 4-5

Directions

1. Add peach slices, sweetener of choice, lemon juice, ice cubes and water in the bowl of your blender and blend on medium speed. Blend another time until smooth.
2. Pour peach drink over ice in glass and garnish with mint leaves and peach slice, if desired.

Nutrition: Calories 99, Fat 0.5 g, Carbs 14.6 g, Protein 2.4 g

Chapter 13:
28-Day Meal Plan to Detox the Liver

Day	Breakfast	Lunch	Dinner
1	Cherry Berry Bulgur Bowl	Tofu Rice	Pomegranate Chicken
2	Baked Curried Apple Oatmeal Cups	Zucchini Cups	Lemon Chicken Mix
3	Healthy Millet Porridge	Black Eyed Peas Stew	Cardamom Chicken and Apricot Sauce
4	Peanut Butter and Cacao Breakfast Quinoa	Herby Chicken Meatloaf	Detox-Liver Arugula and Broccoli Soup
5	Egg and Veggie Muffins	Tilapia With Avocado & Red Onion	Chicken and Spinach Cakes
6	Breakfast Tacos	Grilled Tomatoes Soup	Chicken and Parsley Sauce
7	Vegetable Omelet	Cauliflower Salad	Sage Turkey Mix
8	Buckwheat and Grapefruit Porridge	Green Buddha Bowl	Sage Turkey Mix
9	Raspberry Pudding	Chickpea Alfredo Sauce	Crispy Fish

10	Pineapple, Macha & Beet Chia Pudding	Italian White Bean Soup	Curry Chicken, Artichokes, and Olives
11	Tapioca Pudding	Easy Asparagus Quiche	Yummy Cedar Planked Salmon
12	Banana Pancakes	Herbed Roasted Cod	Zucchini and Mozzarella Casserole
13	Nectarine Pancakes	Lean Mean Soup	Ginger Chicken Drumsticks
14	Pancakes	Avocado Tomato Salad	Miso-Glazed Salmon
15	Peach Muffins	Tofu Spinach Sauté	Lemon Chicken Mix
16	Blueberry Muffins	Chickpea Eggplant Salad	Tuna Noodle Casserole
17	Avocado Spread	Spanish Tomato Salad	Feta and Pesto Wrap
18	Deviled eggs	Garlic Chicken Thigh	Healthy Carrot Ginger Soup
19	Spicy Cucumbers	Smoked Salmon and Watercress Salad	Tasty Lime Cilantro Cauliflower Rice
20	Herbed Spinach Frittata	Lean Mean Soup	Sage Turkey Mix
21	Pumpkin Flax Granola	Crispy Fennel Salad	Turmeric Chicken Soup

22	Broiled Parmesan Avocado	Roasted Green Beans and Mushrooms	Healthy Silky Tortilla Soup
23	Mexican Scrambled Eggs in Tortilla	Extraordinary Green Hummus	Pan Seared Salmon
24	Raspberry Overnight Porridge	Pork Chops and Relish	Healthy Carrot Ginger Soup
25	Turkey and Spinach Scramble on Melba Toast	Grilled Harissa Chicken	Chicken Tortilla Avocado Soup
26	Mexican Style Burritos	Salmon and Corn Salad	Spicy Chicken and Kale
27	Quinoa Bowls With Avocado and Egg	Crockpot Lentil Soup	Tuna Salad
28	Cherry Berry Bulgur Bowl	Arugula and Sweet Potato Salad	Lemon Rosemary Salmon

Measurement Conversion Chart

Volume Equivalents (Liquid)

US Standard	US Standard (ounces)	Metric (approximate)
2 tablespoons	1 fl. oz.	30 mL
¼ cup	2 fl. oz.	60 mL
½ cup	4 fl. oz.	120 mL
1 cup	8 fl. oz.	240 mL
1 ½ cups	12 fl. oz.	355 mL
2 cups or 1 pint	16 fl. oz.	475 mL
4 cups or 1 quart	32 fl. oz.	1 L
gallon	128 fl. oz.	4 L

Volume Equivalents (Dry)

US Standard	Metric (approximate)
⅛ teaspoon	0.5 mL
¼ teaspoon	1 mL
½ teaspoon	2 mL
¾ teaspoon	4 mL
1 teaspoon	5 mL
1 tablespoon	15 mL
¼ cup	59 mL
⅓ cup	79 mL

½ cup	118 mL
⅔ cup	156 mL
¾ cup	177 mL
1 cup	235 mL
2 cups or 1 pint	475 mL
3 cups	700 mL
4 cups or 1 quart	1 L

Oven Temperatures

Fahrenheit (F)	*Celsius (C) (approximate)*
250°F	120°C
300°F	150°C
325°F	165°C
350°F	180°C
375°F	190°C
400°F	200°C
425°F	220°C
450°F	230°C

Weight Equivalents

US Standard	Metric (approximate)
½ ounce	1 g
1 ounce	3 g
2 ounces	6 g
4 ounces	11 g
8 ounces	22 g
12 ounces	34 g
16 ounces or 1 pound	450 g

Conclusion

Thank you for making it to the end of this book. I trust that you have learned a lot about fatty liver disease. The ball is now in your court concerning taking care of your health. Remember, liver disease is not a life sentence, and it can be managed to the point where you enjoy all aspects of your life.

You must take care of yourself by going natural when it comes to the food you eat and including at least 30 minutes of physical exercise every day.

Spread the word to your friends and family, and let us help spread awareness about fatty liver disease, which we need to manage and treat.

Good health is the best gift you can give yourself! All the best!

Printed in Great Britain
by Amazon